STUMBLING BLOCKS TO STEPPING STONES

SHARI LYN RUSCH

To Rochelle, with a song in my heart! God Bless — S— Rusch

ARC
PRESS
Seattle, WA

ARC PRESS
P.O. Box 82627
Kenmore, WA 98028

Cover design: Garth Everett, Advertising Center
Text typesetting & artwork: Advertising Center, Redmond, WA

I dedicate this book to my mother, Lynda Pressey. She gave me life, never ending love and the will to survive. And to my Grandpa, Oscar Eyrikson. He taught me to have pride in myself, that humor was the best cure for pain, and that when I hurt, he could make it rain pennies. I love you both.

FORWARD

The information contained in this book comes from a young lady who has experienced the trauma of an educational system which has been slow to accept, appreciate and acknowledge the fact that learning disabilities do exist and that the children with them can be helped if we as educators are willing to take the time to understand and work with them and not label them as non-educable. The insight that we can all gain from this warm and sometimes heart wrenching book will at times anger you, make you cry, make you laugh, and above all help you become more aware that all children can be helped. For parents, this is a book giving you information about learning disabled children and giving you a clearer understanding and a renewed appreciation for all children. For the educator, it will provide insight into how to deal with learning disabled students, but more importantly it shares the tremendous insights of one who has gone through the system which is under-staffed and under-funded. It is a tribute to those who dedicate their lives to helping all children, regardless of their differences, excel to their greatest potential and are the true definition of the term "Educator." I encourage all those who dedicate their lives to the betterment of our children to read and grow from the information that Shari has provided.

If we take the information within these pages and use it, then we can help all children to see that their limitations can be overcome with encouragement and patience, a virtue which we so often forget. Shari is an inspiration to me and to many who have had the opportunity to come into contact with her. She has been a constant source of motivation to many learning disabled students with whom I have had the pleasure of working during my years as a teacher and school administrator.

With my greatest admiration to Shari and my commitment to the education of all children, I salute Shari for her commitment to the education of the children of America. I sincerely hope and pray that you will use the information within these pages to help you further understand the children you have contact with over the years.

George N. Valison
Principal
Lake Chelan High School

INTRODUCTION

When I was a child, I felt very special. At times I was so bold as to think that God had chosen me to be an angel on earth. That may sound silly but I was a child with an elaborate imagination and a heart that seemed to feel what others couldn't feel, ears that could hear pain and laughter in others' voices, and eyes that could read people's faces before I could ever read the written word. I felt more emotion, more pain, but also more joy than anyone I had ever come into contract with. When you feel that much you also feel responsible to the world. I had the overwhelming sense that if I could only be more in every way to everyone, I could save the world; all the fragile and all the meek. Even as a child I felt chosen - I just didn't know what I was chosen to do.

The feeling of being chosen for a special purpose is something that I think every child has. I was lucky not to have completely lost that feeling as I grew older. However, I didn't just feel special, I was special, unusual, unique, and gifted. Interestingly enough, those words are often used to describe children who have disabilities. I think they are appropriate words, for children who have lost one area of functioning often can do things that others cannot. The difficult thing is to never lose sight of those gifts; to never believe that because we are different, we are wrong.

As you read this book, I hope that you will remember several things. No matter what has happened to me in this life, both bad and good, those experiences have shaped me into the person that I am today. Even harsh words spoken to me in anger or frustration are part of what has made me the strong person that I am. If you are a parent or a teacher you may sometimes find yourself hurting inside as you read my words. It seems that no matter how much I can make you laugh with one of my stories or how many times I pay tribute to those who influenced me so greatly, it is easy to focus attention on the rough spots in my life. Please don't. Realize that the stories in this book were put there for us to learn from together.

I want you all to know that I have searched myself intently as I wrote each word of this book. I have tried mightily to recreate the year by year struggles and triumphs of my life. I have tried to equally balance the sorrow and the joy, and mingle it all with at least some of my ever present humor about the past. Sometimes it was hard to find the humor in a particular experience, but I included even those stories because as I said before, each experience has molded me. I want each reader to know that sometimes both the highs and the lows of my story will touch a chord in you. You might even need to think about what I have said for awhile. That is okay! Sometimes when you hear someone else's story, their pain collides with yours, and it is hard to separate what you feel as you read from what you have experienced personally. When you read about my life, you may have to confront some of the laughter and tears of your own life. I want you to know that I understand your struggle, whatever it may be. I understand how hard it is to get through it. You will. If any part of this book, even the humorous parts, touch a sad chord in you and you need to put the book down for awhile and get hold of you emotions, that is alright. You will come back to it when you can.

I write this introduction because I want teachers to know how much I respect and support them. I am studying to be a teacher myself. I am honored to think that I will one day stand in front of a classroom, to follow in the footsteps of the great teachers I have had in my life. I want my family to know that they have been a great inspiration to me. I want all the kids out there to know that they will rise above the struggle, not just because I did, but because they too have the strength and the talent and are destined to fulfill a great purpose in this life.

From the time I was small, I believed I was chosen. I went through many trials by fire, but I was never alone. Now I realize what I was meant to do. This special, disabled, gifted child was not brought here to save the world, but simply to make a difference, even if it's just a small difference, in the lives of others by sharing her story. Here is my story.

CHAPTER 1

MEETING ADAM

The morning did not start out very well. I ordered my breakfast at 6:30 a.m., and despite several phone calls to the restaurant, by eight o'clock I still hadn't received it. Just as my ride arrived in front of the hotel to take me to my morning assembly, a waitress came running out of the restaurant with my tray. I told her that there was no time to eat breakfast, but she handed me the tray and left without a word. I shrugged my shoulders and went out to catch my ride.

By the time I reached the school where I was to speak, I had finished little of my breakfast. My appetite was lost somewhere between the watery oatmeal and greasy hashbrowns. My juice looked too red to be the cranberry juice I had ordered, but I reached for it and took a big gulp. My "cranberry" juice turned out to be maraschino cherry juice. I swallowed, muttered under my breath, and dropped it in the nearest garbage can. So much for a power breakfast!

When we arrived at the school, I gathered up my briefcase and tape recorder and headed for the administration office to meet the school's activities coordinator and to get instructions on where to go. I waited for several minutes. When the activities coordinator, Mr. Smith, entered the room, I put out my hand to greet him. He mumbled, "Nice to meet you," and led me to the gym.

As we walked, Mr. Smith said, "Don't expect much from these kids. Last time we had an assembly, they all walked out. We haven't had an assembly here for a while because of that." I couldn't help but think, "They walked out? Who allowed that?"

After giving speeches for a couple of years, I had become very sensitive to the feelings of people in each school I visited. This school, like so many others, had a pervasive sense of helplessness permeating from every voice, every face, every classroom. You could almost hear people saying, "So many kids, so many issues, so little time." I felt Mr. Smith looking at me like so many had before him and sensed that he was wondering what a twenty-two year old girl could possibly say that could move these kids? I knew what he was thinking, for I had wondered the same thing many times myself. How could I, just one person, make a difference? I am not a rock band, I am not a multimedia presentation. I am just one person standing on the gymnasium floor. There were times that I, like the educators I met, felt small in the presence of so many kids who needed so much. Somehow God always gave me strength to stand before them and give my message in hopes that at least one might listen.

While the microphones were being set up, the kids in the audience were getting restless and loud. My hands were shaking so hard

1

that I began wishing my dress had some pockets that I could hide them in. My introduction was made and I took the stage. The kids continued to talk and make noise despite the fact that I had begun my speech. I paused for just a moment, took a deep breath, gripped the microphone in my right hand as hard as possible and put my feet a couple of inches apart, as if to brace myself for a forceful hit.

I started talking again. At first, the noise level in that gym didn't go down. In fact, it probably got louder. But I kept talking. The minute I said, "Looking at me now it may be hard to believe, but at one time I was told I would probably not progress in school much further than the fifth or sixth grade," they began to listen. I continued, "This was because I was born with learning disabilities and I couldn't do the very things that many of you take for granted. Do I look different to you? Would you call me names if you passed me on the street? Probably not, because now the glasses and the lisp are gone. My learning disabilities are hidden away in my head. I can walk down any street or hallway and no one would know the difference. That is how far I have come in my life. But what about all the other people in this world who can't transform, who can't hide their differences? Do they deserve any less than I? I can fit in now, but I still remember what it was like to be called different, stupid, ugly, lazy, retarded, reject and four eyes." The noise in the gym had stopped. For the rest of the assembly, the young people listened attentively to my story. They laughed with me, some even cried with me. At the end they stood to applaud.

I began my speech feeling frightened, but I was unwilling to back down. In the end, I won their respect. I refused to give up in hopes that one person might hear. And I got my wish. I met many kids that day, more than I can remember. But one young man's face will be ingrained in my memory forever.

MY NAME IS ADAM

He stood in the crowd of people that surrounded me after the assembly. He waited patiently. Each time I turned to him, he waved me on to another person. He waited until the whole crowd was gone and we were the only two people left in the gym. Finally, he raised up his eyes to look at me. His tear-stained face was becoming wet again. I told him, "It's okay, take your time," and I put my arm around him.

It was obvious from his first words that he had a speech impediment of some kind. His jaw didn't seem to move the way it should to enable him to make the sounds necessary for speech. I leaned a little closer so that I could hear what he was saying. He said softly, "My name is Adam and I need help."

I knelt down to look him in the eyes and said, "How can I help you?" What a question!

Adam and I walked to the classroom where I was to meet with just the learning disabled students, as I always do following my assemblies. It was at this time that Adam told me his story. He was originally from Calcutta, India. When he was very young, his father died in a construction accident and he was left with his brother and mother. He left home one day to find his mother, who was working in the city, but he couldn't find her nor could he tell anyone where he lived. Adam was turned over to an agency for lost children and was eventually adopted by an American family.

When I met him, Adam was struggling to try to learn English. His speech impediment slowed his progress, and his dark skin color set him even further apart from the other students in this predominantly white school. His coat sleeves hung down on his hands and his jeans were worn and out of style.

He had a learning disability, but he did not know what kind. All he did know was that he was having a terrible time in school. With all of his needs, somehow he was overlooked.

I put my arm around Adam as we walked, and thought to myself, "What is his most important problem right now?" I asked him, "Are you in a speech therapy class?" He shook his head no. "What about a resource room for learning disabled students?" He wasn't sure. When we got to the resource room, the teacher didn't seem to recognize him and he didn't recognize her. I got the feeling he had never been in this room.

I answered questions from all the students in the class, while Adam sat quietly at the back of the room with his books stacked in front of him. As I spoke with the students the resource room teacher, who looked very tired, leaned up against her desk.

When the class was over and I had said good-bye to all of the students, I went back to Adam and said, "Come on, let's go see if we can get you some help." He nodded, and I took his hand and led him over to the resource room teacher. As he stood there with me, he started to cry again.

I said, "This is Adam." She still looked at him as though she had never seen him before. "He came up to me after the assembly and said that he needs help in school. He told me that he is not in a speech therapy program. Can you tell me why?" She said, "He doesn't qualify." In my mind I am thinking, "What do you have to do to qualify, not be able to speak at all?" She shook her head in agreement with the expression I unknowingly had on my face. She continued, "Adam, whose class are you in?" He looked confused but he rattled off a couple of names and she nodded her head.

I said, "He needs help. I don't want to leave until I find someone who is willing to work with him." She looked weary when I said this and although she didn't verbalize it, her look said, "Shari, I want to help him and all of the other children at this school. I wish I could help them all." She took a pad of paper, wrote his name down, and placed it on her desk.

I knew I had just put another weight on her shoulders, but if a resource room teacher couldn't help, who could? Where else could Adam go?

When I asked why Adam hadn't been able to get help for his problems, she responded, "Shari, he is just one of many children who slip through the cracks." I looked at Adam, who was crying even harder now. I knew why, for I could not count the number of times that I had slipped through the cracks, slipped through the system, slipped through the hands of those who were unsure what to do with me.

I hugged Adam tightly and I thanked the teacher for her time. I started to walk out the door and caught a glimpse of Adam's name on that pad of paper. I could only hope that once I left she would find the resources and the energy to help him.

Adam and I are alike in many ways. We are just two of the millions of school age children and adults who are afflicted with learning disabilities. Sometimes hidden, sometimes visible, our differences vary from slight to extreme. Some people can make it through life almost unaffected by their challenges. With a slight alteration in how they respond towards their environment, the problem for them can be almost nonexistent. However, for most like Adam and me, our disabilities will be obvious to others and to ourselves for as long as we live.

But does that have to mean a death sentence? A wasted life? No, it doesn't. With patience and understanding, learning disabled children and adults can make it. With the use of alternative forms of learning, people with learning disabilities can go on to become successful, independent adults. Without those simple things, it is hard to say what will happen to us.

We often possess high intelligence with above average IQs, but there is a difference in our brain that makes it difficult and sometimes impossible to learn in the traditional way. If no alternative forms of learning are provided, it is likely that we will feel completely defeated in education. We will drop out, be kicked out, hate ourselves, hate others for not understanding, become self-destructive, or destroy the people and things around us. The energy, the frustration, and the anger goes somewhere. It can either go into alternative forms of learning and functioning, or it can go into self-hate.

Statistics show that our jails, institutions for juvenile delinquency, and other correctional facilities have a high percentage of learning disabled people in their populations. What does this mean? Are learning disabled people bad? Are they born criminals? Not at all. They are simply people who have struggled to learn to survive in a society that prizes education, yet doesn't fund its schools properly. A society which says that different is not acceptable, and that success is the only way to find acceptance. The problem is that there are few alternatives provided for those who have a difference or handicap to help them achieve that success, and ultimately acceptance.

In short, people have three basic needs: love, acceptance, and a purpose in life. If we don't find acceptance in the mainstream, we will look elsewhere. If kids can't get in with the brains, the jocks, or the cheerleaders at their school, where do they go? The parking lot crowd? The stoners (drug users)? The pushers? It's amazing what people will do to be loved - even steal, cheat, or lie. If given the proper avenue for their energy and skills, this would not happen.

From childhood on, we are told to line up, walk straight, be quiet, sit still. What if you can't clearly see all that is around you? What if your hearing is not impaired but seems to be muffled? What if you find it hard to concentrate because of noise, movement or color? What if you are hyperactive and don't know how to focus your energy? What if you look at a book, but you cannot read the written word, put meaning to a symbol, or sound to a letter? What if the words jump all over the page uncontrollably? What if right and left, north, south, east and west mean nothing to you?

Can you imagine being like this? At every turn someone asks why you don't try harder? All the while you want to do better, but feel helpless against your challenges. If you experienced these things, would you make it through high school? Would you think attending college was a possibility?

What if you could be successful in school using another form of learning, but few knew how to teach you those alternatives, or were aware that those alternatives existed? What if at every turn those around you said or implied, "If you don't do it like everyone else, you aren't smart, right and good"? How would that make you feel? It usually makes children feel that they should learn in that one traditional way that doesn't work for them. This effort is misdirected and will ultimately lead to failure. Each failure leads them closer and closer to the belief that they are stupid, dumb, unteachable, and untalented. Every talent, academic or otherwise, any motivation to try, is lost amid an enormous sense of failure. What they really need to do is to learn in a way that works best for them.

There was a time when few people wanted to deal with a disabled student in their classroom. There was a time when all students who were different were removed from the "normal." Look at how far we have come. We no longer institutionalize, we integrate. I know, sometimes it doesn't work perfectly. But I give anyone a round of applause for being innovative, for trying any possible way to open up the doors of every classroom, and embrace the diversity in all students, including those with specific challenges and disabilities.

I so am encouraged to see that more educators - not just resource room teachers - are becoming equipped to deal with learning disabled students in the mainstream classroom. At first it must seem like just another mountain to climb in an already staggering load of work. But the results from your efforts are young people, like myself, who emerge from schools with a sense of self esteem, confidence, and the ability to maneuver in a world which does not provide a resource room to help us.

I believe that every teacher must be educated about learning disabilities, and given the proper support and resources to not only learn to detect students who have specific learning disabilities, but to teach them in the mainstream classroom. Without the proper education and experience in learning disabilities, teachers cannot be expected to recognize these problems and deal with them effectively.

I think it is hard to realize why integration is so important unless you have seen what happens to kids who have been separated. The main problem with the "resource room" concept is not about what they do, for they provide support and a foundation of skills and help that will support that child through the education process. It is about what they imply. When a child is diagnosed and then receives help through a resource room, there is often a sense of doom involved with that form of intervention. Parents and children often feel that they have hit a wall, that this is a dead-end in terms of education. Separation in any shape or form is more painful than I can express in words, both to children and to parents. Anything that we can do to alleviate the stigma, the pain, and the embarrassment associated with being disabled and/or different will make a world of difference for the children and the families who are a part of the special education system.

Even if no accurate time line can be given, it is so important that children see the resource room as a launching pad, a place for them to improve their skills over a period of time. The ultimate goal is to return to the mainstream when they are ready. There must be a goal to motivate them to move forward. If the child feels that there is no hope, they will no longer try. Without a goal in mind, a child enters the system but is soon transformed into a "resource kid," with all the self-esteem and behavior problems that go with that label.

6

To fully understand the issues that face learning disabled students, we must look at the educators who teach them. There are many wonderful and highly qualified resource room teachers. But these teachers, like most educators, not only work with limited resources, they also face a pervasive lack of compassion from others, who look at their students as being a waste of time to try and teach. Their job at times is devalued, because some people don't realize the potential that exists in learning disabled children. Unfortunately they are often met by a teacher or administrator who is just fed up with a kid who is struggling with all aspects of academics, and as a result of this struggle is a constant source of behavior problems. Because they are overworked and/or possibly don't understand why the child acts out in such a way, they give up in frustration and hand the kid back to the resource room teacher. While others give up in frustration, a resource room teacher must look after a full load of children who are all facing these same problems. Resource room teachers are also met by parents who are at their wits end, frustrated and angry for their children, and at those who are supposed to have the answers, but don't. All the while, the stigma on them and their students becomes greater. They, like their students, suffer under the stigma caused by the system of separation.

The route to the resource room usually involves diagnosing, testing and labeling. These steps are the route that schools must take to receive the funding that is necessary for the education of special needs students under the current laws. All of these are good functions, but it is also a safety factor. If the child is labled and placed, it is a chapter closed in the education life of the child. Everyone feels good because the child needs are being met, but are they? Labeling may provide an effective way to sort kids according to their needs, but that system cannot offset the emotional impact the child feels as a result of being separated. Imagine how it feels for a kid who has to walk down the hall into Room 11 when all his peers are saying, "Only dummies go to that room. Are you dumb? Retarded? You just don't fit in with us!"

My question has always been, just exactly who is benefiting from this? Separate is not equal and it never will be! The real result is that the learning disabled person's anger and frustration over being different, and the stigma that is attached to being a resource room kid, grows into rage at themselves and others. Some will fight their way out of the resource room into the mainstream and go on to be successful. They look and perform just like everyone else, but no one knows what it really takes for them to compete. Some kill themselves or have nervous breakdowns in the process.

Others will disrupt class; yell, scream and generally be impossible to deal with until the teacher kicks them out, which is just what some of these students want. Then they can sit in the office and don't have to learn how to read. These students are called troublemakers. People come to expect them to act in a certain way and they fulfill those expectations. Very few people have the time to find out why these kids act the way they do. The kids like it better this way anyway. They get attention from somebody (it may be negative but it is better than no attention) and they are known as the bad kid rather than learning disabled. They have made a "reputation," a place for themselves. Anything becomes better than being called stupid.

There is still one other scenario. It's the kids who just sit there. Somebody looked at them at some point and said in an ominous voice, "I'm sorry. You have a learning disability." From that point on, everyone believed that child was not going to be successful. Maybe no one explained that you don't die from a learning disability, maybe there were no answers given, only big words for a problem that nobody can see and few understand. Maybe, like so many, this student was never diagnosed or was diagnosed so late that he has already begun to believe that learning and success are impossible. "I try and I fail. If I don't try, I won't have to fail." So they sit there. Some are passed on to the next grade. People say, "They aren't bad kids, they just don't try." The people who pass them without proper help or skill levels think they are helping the child. But no one benefits when these children grow up and graduate from high school without knowing how to read!

Another alternative is to hold learning disabled students back a year so that they can mature. The idea makes sense. Give these children an opportunity to catch up. The problem is that being held back means you are different. Being different is not okay when you are the child being held back. Some kids will survive it, others will die inside with the weight of the embarrassment and the weight of knowing that repeating a class means another year of school added to their sentence. At some point it crosses their minds, "If I don't get it this year, will they just keep holding me back? Will I be in third grade forever?" Again, without proper help and alternative learning methods, it is hard to say how long a student will stay at the third grade level before he is either passed on, pushed through, or best of all, receives the services that will help him succeed.

I hope it is clear to you now that I empathize with all that parents, teachers, administrators, and kids face when dealing with learning disabilities and the issues that surround them. There is no easy answer, but there is common ground.

If Adam's story took place fifty years ago and we were examining the situation today, everyone would say, "See, look how we have changed." The truth is, I met Adam only three years ago and I still meet others like him every day. We have come a long way, but we have a long way to go. The strides we have made in all areas of society are minuscule in comparison to the number of people with learning disabilities.

Now some of you may be saying to yourself, "But this doesn't affect me." When people drop out, commit suicide, commit crimes as a means to survive, or drink and take drugs to hide the pain of failure, it is a problem that affects all of us!

Our tax dollars build the schools and the prisons. My question is, what do we prefer to invest in, education or delinquency? When people don't make it, when people ask for help and don't get it, we all lose. We lose a potential tax payer, a potential citizen who could make a difference in this world. That is a loss to us all.

We as a nation cannot allow children to slip unnoticed through any system of society. It is up to all of us to realize that the future lies within our children. We all have a vested interest in supporting schools and other programs which help kids become successful adults.

I fight now for this cause because I know that it was by the grace of God that I had a chance in this life and I didn't end up on the streets, in prison, or as one of the many functionally illiterate in our society. A loving mother, supportive teachers, and my own determination enabled me to survive a childhood with learning disabilities and a life filled with challenges. I am a veteran of this fight and I am only twenty-five years old.

My story started the day I was born. I came into this world with a 75 percent vision loss in my right eye and a 25 percent vision loss in my left eye. I was a sickly, hyperactive child who spoke with a lisp, and I had a whole host of audio, visual and motor disabilities. At home I was able to find peace and understanding for my differences. Outside my home, school and society had little tolerance for my problems. I became an outcast simply because I was different.

A person who started out as a happy, carefree child was soon transformed into a child who hated school and herself because she couldn't fit in or learn in the way that other kids could.

By the end of my first grade year, my parents were told that I would probably never go beyond the fifth or sixth grade level and that I should be taken out of the public school system and put in an institution with others like me. Because of the day and age, there was a lack of knowledge regarding students like myself. It was not uncommon for people to look at a child like me and feel that I was unteachable. It happened then and sometimes still does.

But where do you go? I was not developmentally disabled. The area where we lived had no special schools for learning disabled children. Anyway, we didn't have the money for one. So where was I supposed to go to school? There was no answer.

But I didn't leave. My mom fought for me to stay in the public schools rather than be separated from the mainstream. She believed in me enough to ask a teacher at our school to keep me in her class for second and third grade. The teacher agreed. I owe a great deal of thanks to Miss Driscoll, for she took time with me, cared about me, talked to me in a soft voice, and looked at me when she spoke. All of a sudden, the classroom became a less frightening and confusing place. It was with her that I began to learn.

Somehow I passed along from grade to grade. Eventually after years of failure and hiding, I developed my own alternative forms of learning that helped me to survive in school and in life. These learning styles were different than what I had first been taught, but then I was different.

I went far beyond the fifth grade. Using my alternative forms of learning, I graduated fourth in my high school class and went on to attend the University of Washington. Yet today, I remember when I was a "slip through the cracks kid." I have gone through the pain and the anguish of feeling that I could never make it in this life. I grew up hiding behind my books so that people would think I was reading, while listening to my friends talk about the book so I wouldn't have to read it; sitting in the back of the room so no one would call on me; being nice and quiet so I could pass on into the next grade.

Spending your whole life hiding is a tiring process. There is always a fear that you might reveal your secret, that someone might find you out. You want to hide, to shut yourself away where nothing can touch you. Away from a world that overwhelms you to such a degree that you feel you will never be able to cope. And yet you see other people achieving their goals and you ask yourself, "Why can't I do those very same things? Why can't I get what I want out of life?" It is then that you have three choices. Either completely give up and do nothing, cheat and lie to get through, or begin one of the hardest fights of your life-trying to succeed despite your learning problems.

I cannot accept that only some people are meant to make it in this life. My own story proves that it is possible. We didn't have money or special tutors and schools. I grew up in a single parent household, with a working mother. I am a product of the public school system and of a life that is not unlike a majority of the kids that I meet everyday.

Children like myself need alternative forms of learning that can be implemented in the mainstream classroom and basic skills that will help them survive in this world. They need to have their challenges understood for what they are: a challenge - not a sentence for a unsuccessful life. They can be successful even with a learning disability. Most of all, they need integration, not separation.

I tell this story to enlighten, to share with you the nameless faces of those who didn't understand me. More importantly are the precious people who did, like my mom who saw the greatness in me, and wonderful teachers, like Miss Driscoll and my first grade resource room teacher, who took the time to teach me. This is a book of hope for all learning disabled people, and all parents and teachers of children with learning problems. But more than that, it is a book about life. It is a journey through years of school experiences, some sad and some joyous. It is also a journey through life challenges like family problems, divorce, suicide, and addiction. This book is about learning to laugh at what used to be painful, and making positive choices in life; it's about learning to do more than just survive, it is about learning to live.

STUMBLING BLOCKS TO STEPPING STONES

CHAPTER 2

Sometimes moms and dads are the only ones who can see the potential Picasso in the colorful finger painting that comes home from kindergarten, or the prima ballerina who shuffles and fumbles across the stage at the ballet recital. Seeing the possibilities in children helps plant the seeds of greatness.

When someone believes in you, it's amazing what you can do, what fears you can overcome, what risks you can take. When someone sees the greatness in you, it's easier to see it in yourself.

When I was little, my mom saw the greatness in me. When I stumbled, and when no one else believed in me, she did. She could look beyond my failures to what I could be. She refused to let the assessments and labels stop her from believing that there was a chance for me.

It was easy for her to be over-protective because she wanted to shelter me from the failures. She protected me, but she also knew when to let go, when the fight needed to be mine. She allowed me to venture beyond her loving arms, beyond her fears so that I might learn to find my own way.

I have heard people say that without my mom I wouldn't have made it. She insists that it was my choices and my determination that allowed me to reach goals others never dreamed were possible. The truth is, she helped me and I learned to help myself. It was my choice, but I don't know how I would have made it without her love.

Being the parent of a child who is different for whatever reason is very hard. I hope that the frustrations and fears that you and your child are experiencing will be lessened by hearing how one mother dealt with the uphill battle of having a different child. In this chapter I have asked my mom, Lynda Pressey, to introduce the child that I used to be.

Shari and I agreed on the importance of this chapter long ago. We both felt that this book needed to address the three most important audiences dealing with this issue: parents, educators, and kids. I have tried several times to start this chapter, only to wind up surrounded by wads of crumpled paper. I wanted to speak to all those who may feel alone in their struggle, but having been through this myself, I found it hard to go back in time and relive the pain of raising a child with special needs.

Today I am happily married, I have a lovely home, a thriving business, and two successful daughters. I look at Shari and I am in awe. She has come so far and accomplished so much. It is much easier to believe that it was always this way than to reach back into the past. For when you reach back, you not only see the accomplishments of your children and yourself, but often you see the pitfalls, the times when you wanted to make everything better for your children but couldn't, the times when you needed a solution for a problem that was bigger than your title as a parent, but couldn't find one.

For most of the years that I was raising Shari I was a single, working mother without a college education, and without the money to provide special schools, tutors, and materials for my child. I did the very best that I could with what I had. I call it the "Fly by the Seat of Your Pants" approach to parenting. No book was there to tell me what to do, so I made it up as I went along. I loved her with everything that I had; I taught her all that I knew so that she would be capable of caring for herself. I praised her for even the smallest things, and when she cried, I cried with her. I couldn't begin to count the times that Shari and I sat huddled together after another day at school that had gone wrong. We sat there until the tears subsided and then we would find something to do together. We would laugh a little and somehow the pain didn't seem so bad.

Don't worry about all the things you don't have - all the resources and skills that some book, television program, or well-meaning person says you need to be a parent - and go with what you have right now. Believe me, the smallest of things can make any child, and especially a child who has challenges, rise above the labels and assessments and become all that you dream they can be.

I grew up at a time when no one had ever spoken the words "learning disability." If you were slow or didn't seem to understand something, you were either "retarded" or a dunce, and stood a meager chance of escaping that assessment. In the latter case, school officials put a dunce cap on your head and put you in the corner until you had learned your lesson. Not the classroom lesson, but a lesson none the less. I was notorious for being either the dunce or the class clown. I learned that if I made people laugh, they often forgot that I wasn't learning. Having a sense of humor, although often directed at myself, got me through high school and graduation no worse for the wear, but without the skills to function at a college level or even with the basic skills to function in life.

Fortunately for me, my mother and father had started me in dancing and musical instrument lessons at a very early age and I had natural singing ability. We dropped the musical instrument part of the lessons when it was discovered that I couldn't read music to save my life and I was playing everything by ear. However, the dancing lessons continued and I prospered. Singing and dancing was my life, and combined with my sense of humor, they made me feel that I was somebody. Being in talent shows at school, or traveling with a USO or Vaudeville troop made me forget, at least for a moment, that I couldn't spell.

During all the time that I was growing up, I never knew that

14

I was learning disabled. Of course, I was aware that words moved and swirled around on the page when I tried to read. Numbers would reverse themselves, but I didn't know why. The fact that I couldn't read music, or understand directions like north, south, east, and west were all manifestations of a condition that actually had a name. That name wasn't "dunce", it was "dyslexia" and other undiagnosed learning disabilities. Because I didn't know that I was learning disabled, I felt incapable in many areas. I often felt, as Shari did, that I didn't fit in. Life moved too fast, and although I was capable in many ways, there were areas of life that scared me to death. Banks, driving a car, and other systems of the world that so many take for granted were very intimidating. At the same time, I knew that I couldn't be the class clown all my life. I knew that to function in the world, I would either have to do it myself and risk failure, or find someone to help me.

As most women of my generation did, at age 21 I got married. When I married I had a high school diploma, but no drivers license. Even with all my alternative talents, I was helpless in some very necessary elements of life. I was forced to depend on people because of my disability. Roger was a man with many wonderful qualities, but I often wonder if I got married thinking that my husband would take care of me. This is a dangerous way to live. What if something should happen to him? Then what?

Our marriage was good. Roger directed our lives, and that is exactly how I thought things should be. According to the prescription of the times, we had it all. He worked, went to night school and was an up-and-coming business man in our community. Although I reversed every key on the typewriter and had no skills in clerical work, I landed a job as a secretary. I took three buses to get to work each day, and managed to have the house clean and dinner on the table by the time my husband got home. Sounds perfect doesn't it?

Our life continued to move upward over the first four years of our marriage. We bought our first house, Roger was working his way up in banking, and after four years of marriage, we were pleased to find out that we were having our first child.

Shawn was bright eyed, full of life, and was such an easy baby to care for that life seemed limitless because of her. With her shining black hair, big brown eyes and olive skin, she was a beautiful child; and she was a bright child. She gave me many opportunities to boast about her advanced development.

Approximately one year later, I found out that I was pregnant again, and I looked forward to the birth of my second child. I had an easy pregnancy and expected that things would be as smooth as they had been with Shawn.

On January 21, 1966, Shari Lyn Rusch, was born in an easy

delivery. The only complication during the delivery process was that she was born with the cord wrapped around her neck, which starved her brain for oxygen, resulting in her head being blue. This is not uncommon. In fact, a similar situation had occurred with Shawn. Although I was alarmed, they unwrapped the cord from her neck, the normal color returned to her face, and the doctor said she would be fine. Although I don't believe that being born a "blue baby" caused Shari's difficulties, more and more research indicates that it can be one of the many possible causes or influencing factors in regards to learning disabilities. I know all of this now, but at the time all I saw was a pretty little blond with dimples so deep that the nurses would tickle her chin just to see her smile.

But Shari didn't smile very much when we brought her home from the hospital. In fact she cried constantly. First, she was not a comfortable baby. It seemed to hurt her when I held her close. If held in the wrong way, she would scream with pain. Because of the way she had lain in the womb before birth, her back was not adjusting well to being moved, so I had to hold her head away from me, support her back, and keep her tiny feet tucked into my chest. Second, she came home from the hospital with what would prove to be the first of many colds. Her back hurt, she was sick, and she cried all the time. Shawn was less than happy with this new bundle of noise and soon asked if we could take her back.

I tried not to compare Shari and Shawn, but the contrast between my two daughters became more apparent every day. Except for minor childhood sniffles and sneezes, Shawn remained healthy and continued to be very advanced for her age. Shari, on the other hand, was always sick and her development seemed very slow.

Eventually Shari's back problem worked itself out and it became a little easier to hold her, but she didn't seem to move through the simple stages of rolling and sitting up like Shawn did. Like a turtle, if Shari was laid on her back she couldn't seem to roll back over again. Not knowing what else to do, I worked with Shari to help her roll and move through these simple steps, but I was growing more and more concerned about her.

Concerns about her physical development were quickly brushed aside when, at three months of age, Shari developed dangerously high, unexplained fevers up to 105.5 degrees accompanied with uncontrollable diarrhea. As the fever's cause was unknown, each time we rushed to the hospital the staff did what they could to treat the symptoms. Along with the fluids that were forced into her fever-wracked body, Shari was dosed with every antibiotic and fever suppressant known to modern medicine at that time. One harrowing night when her temperature reached almost 106, the physicians told us that they did not expect her to live. Though not certain of the cause of her illness, they felt that Shari's immune system was deficient and they began experimental treatments with gamma globulin. Though the treatments proved unsuccessful in supplying Shari with good health, she did survive that night.

Eventually Shari's health problems stabilized and she managed to get through her first year, but chronic colds, sniffles, and ear infections would become a normal part of her life from that time forward. Years later, we would learn that much of Shari's health problems were related to severe food allergies which went undiagnosed. She spit up milk, so they put her on soy based formula. We now know that she is even more allergic to soy than milk. Her health went up and down depending on what foods she ate - I didn't know what to do. When she was a baby, nobody ever said that you could be <u>that</u> allergic to food!

Still worrying about her health, I also focused on her physical development. Like everything else, Shari finally learned to turn over and move around more successfully, she just did it in a different way than most children. For instance, Shari developed her own special style of locomotion, an elbow-only crawl. Instead of combining her arms and legs to move, she just dragged herself around on her elbows. Then at 14 months old, Shari began to walk. Fourteen months is not an unusual age for those first steps, but it seemed that by moving from her dragging, elbow-only style of crawling to walking, that she may have skipped some important developmental steps along the way.

More disturbing than her physical development was her intellectual development. She often sat in front of the television for hours rocking herself in a repetitive pattern. Not only did she rock in a repetitive way, but she tended to repeat small words like "Mama," "Da-da," and other early beginnings of speech over and over again. As a child and as an adult, Shari has taught herself that comfort can be found in patterns and organization. Her thoughts are scattered and her brain is overwhelmed, so she calms herself by using patterns and organizational skills. I know this now, but at the time I didn't understand this funny little kid who rocked, repeated in repetition, and was disrupted and upset by anything that changed her pattern.

She was alert and mobile just like any one and a half year old, but her processes, the way that she did things seemed either delayed, or mixed up. It took her longer to reach each level of development.

I often felt overwhelmed and afraid in the face of Shari's problems. From doctors, to relatives, so many people had so many opinions, but few had any answers for what was wrong and how to treat her. I felt torn between trying to be a wife and mother, and at the same time, dealing with the overwhelming question of what will happen to Shari.

Although I had been doing volunteer work throughout the first years of Shawn's and Shari's lives, Roger suggested that with my experience in show business I open my own business. I was a little reluctant, but he set out to find a building, a contractor, and other requirements for starting my own modeling agency. I set out to find a baby-sitter for our daughters.

I not only felt guilty about beginning a career when my girls were so young, I was particularly worried about anyone who would be caring for Shari. She needed someone who was sensitive and understanding. I vowed that I would not sign any papers for the business until I found the perfect person to watch over my kids. Mrs. Sager came like an answer to a prayer. Having raised a large family of her own, she was certainly qualified to love and care for Shawn and Shari. She cooked just like my mom, the old-fashioned way with good seasonings-mashed potatoes, penny circle carrots, and fried chicken that was browned outside and tender inside. I felt blessed to have found this wonderful woman to take care of my children. I was ready to begin my business.

Not long after I began to work, Shari's fevers started again. The doctors were at a loss to know what to do for her. The continued gamma globulin treatments weren't working. A friend told me that the doctors who discovered the immune deficiency ailment and gamma globulin treatment were at the University of Washington in Seattle. I made an appointment. Shari was tested and re-tested. She was not a candidate for the treatment and, in fact, it was very dangerous for her. The University physicians recommended that Shari be seen by two physicians in West Seattle who found that Shari had severe allergies to grass, dust, and an assortment of various other things (Shari's food allergies were not diagnosed at this time, however.) Under their care, she began to show some improvement.

Despite the improvements in Shari's health, other problems continued. While we had spent many hours at the hospital during her infancy for fevers, now we visited often with injuries. She was described as "an accident looking for a place to happen." I assumed Shari just had more than her share of typical toddler falls. One time period particularly stands out in my memory. Shari fell against our Boston rocking chair, cutting an exact imprint of the end of the chair into her forehead. We were off to the hospital for stitches. Just a few days later, she placed her hand on a stove burner causing third degree burns, even though she had been cautioned by a sitter not to touch the burner. Another trip to the emergency room. Two days later, as I held her "good" hand, we waded together in Puget Sound. Shari cried, "Ow-ee, Toe-ie," and pointed to her toes but could give no further explanation for her distress. When I picked her up, her tiny little feet were cut to ribbons. Off we went to the emergency room again!

Shari made it to her third birthday. At three years of age, she could say only a few understandable words and a gibberish that only Shawn and a couple of others could understand. That fall Roger and I visited California, leaving Shawn with friends and Shari with my parents. The separation was good for Shari, who was forced to communicate more clearly since her translator, Shawn, was not present. When we returned from the trip, we saw what could only be described as a miracle. Shari spoke much more clearly and increased her ability to construct sentences. They were peppered with a stutter and a lisp, but the sentences made sense. We could hardly believe it and were grateful that she could finally talk. The falls continued, but she was healthier and was communicating more successfully.

Just before Christmas that year, a traumatic event provided the beginnings of insight into Shari's problems. Shari was with me on a shopping trip to buy a last minute Christmas gift. Shari was tired and wanted to lay on my lap and sleep. I did not fasten her seat belt. As I pulled into an intersection, a car without lights came out of nowhere at break-neck speed. The impact was so hard my car became airborne, turned in a full circle and landed in a parking lot facing the opposite direction. Shari lay in a crumpled ball at my feet and there was little left of the front of my car.

I hurt all over, but I picked up the bloody bundle that resembled my child. Smoke was pouring from the engine, and some kids helped us get out of the car. Both Shari and I were in shock; but as usual, I was concerned with details and my mind raced. I gave orders with phone numbers— call our doctor, call our home, don't let Shawn see us in this condition, tell Roger where we are. We were bloody and waiting for an ambulance. Four girls were hurt in the other car. The driver and the other male passenger fled the scene on foot, but they left behind their open bottles of alcohol.

When only one ambulance arrived, they were going to stack us in like fire wood. I refused to go, and insisted that Roger drive us himself and that he go by our house and get Shari's blanket first. Somehow we made it to the hospital.

Shari's face looked horrible, and the doctor rushed her into surgery right away. The cut on her forehead extended through her eyelid and another cut went along the base of her eyelashes. I had bruises, a broken rib, lumps on my head and legs, and a concussion. I wanted to stay with Shari that night, but Roger was concerned about my condition and made me go home. I was awake all night worrying about Shari, all alone in the hospital.

Our family made a sad holiday display that Christmas. I felt like a steamroller had rolled over the top of me and I wore a neck brace along with my bruises. My mother was in a car accident

19

in November and was in a back and neck brace. Shari's face was black and blue and she had a patch over her eye. My sister, Pam, was in the middle of cancer treatment and not doing very well. I don't remember what foods were served or what presents were exchanged except for walking dolls for the girls and a cart for Shari. But I remember Shari saying in her lisping speech, "I can't thee my prethenths." I thought it had to do with the bandages.

Shari healed quickly and her black and blue face returned to normal. Three months after the accident, I took Shari to a noted eye surgeon in Seattle to determine if the accident caused any permanent damage to her sight. She looked very tiny sitting in the adult chair in his examining room. The nurse came in holding a chart filled with boats, balls, cars and other objects easily identified by children. She pointed to the top of the chart, and Shari said, "boat." The nurse then pointed at the second picture. Shari turned away and said, "That's too hard for me." I gave her one of my "mom looks," for she could be a tease. I thought she just didn't want to play this game. The nurse covered her other eye, pointed at the boat again, and Shari, turning her head, said, "That's too hard." My "mom look" became a little more pronounced. The nurse went out into the hall to confer with the doctor. I will never forget what I overheard her say. "That child is nearly blind, doctor. She can see the top figure with one eye and nothing with the other." I could then hear only indistinguishable mumblings and my eyes burned with tears. It began to make sense. I began to take potshots at my ability as a mother. How could I have been so blind to her blindness. The falls, the mistakes, the accidents, her lack of common sense about any kind of imminent danger. The near miss when our neighbor grabbed her from in front of a speeding car as she toddled behind Roger and didn't seem to see the car about to hit her.

The doctor came in to talk to me. I was afraid, but asked point blank, "How blind is she?" He answered, "She was born with 75 percent blindness in one eye and 25 percent blindness in the other." My next question was, "Can she be helped?" He said, "Yes, she can be helped, and she will be able to see much better than she can now." I heard other words, too. Amblyopia, astigmatism, tunnel vision, ability to define shapes. I was afraid, but I was ready to do whatever was necessary. Surgery? Glasses? I wanted to fix it and make it well. So the process began - years of glasses, therapy, eye patches, drops and medicines and more things which often helped her vision, but did nothing for her self-esteem.

When Shari was four years old, I realized that everything she touched seemed to have disaster connected to it. I often went to sleep at night wondering what was going to happen to this child. I felt that if I didn't offer her encouragement, she probably would feel so badly about herself that she wouldn't go on. It was then that I began looking for things, anything that I could teach Shari an then praise her for. I thought of everything and anything that might be of help in building Shari's self-confidence. Her coordination was poor, but water was soothing to her. I taught her to wash dishes and bought her a dish rack and a stool for her to stand on. She spent hours washing dishes, only to drain the sink and wash them over again.

I also purchased plastic dishes and glasses after the first week of teaching her how to clear the table. Shari carried the dishes with great care; but her height was at odds with the height of the sink, resulting in breakage and tears. Bed making came next, followed by dusting, mopping, and anything else that might help Shari feel better about herself and become an independent person. Shawn picked up all these skills with ease, but they were not the center of her life as they were in Shari's. Shawn was popular, had a growing circle of activities, and possessed a wealth of self-assurance.

The comparisons between Shawn and Shari came and went from every direction. The gaps in skill levels between the two were obvious and kids and adults often said hurtful things which fell hard on Shari. It was difficult for Shawn because although it feels good to be complimented, when it is at the expense of your sister, it is hard to know how to handle it. It also left Shawn feeling the burden of either wanting to protect Shari from the other kids at school and in the neighborhood, or disassociating herself from Shari so that she, too, wouldn't be made fun of. It is a terrible role for any child to be in. Whatever Shawn touched turned to gold. Shari's successes earned personal gold stars from me, but little accolade from the world at large.

Spring 1970 held considerable sadness for both me and Roger. On May 30, my sister Pam died after a six and a half year battle with cancer. A month later, Roger lost his job in the savings and loan industry. As second vice-president of a three-branch company, he was a rising star. However, he discovered the illegal acts his fellow officers were committing, and when he refused to play along, he was fired. It hit him like a ton of bricks. Following these events, our marriage began a downward plunge, and we just couldn't get it back together.

Soon after Pam died, friends called to say their beach house was for sale. They knew we loved it, so they offered us a great buy. Though we really couldn't afford it, the offer was just too good to refuse. It turned out to be a grand place to heal.

The girls and I spent as much of the next nine summers there as possible. The beach provided the serenity, peace and joy that can be found in only a few places on this earth. Shawn and Shari

21

marched in the Kiddie Parade in the local fair, and entered every piece of art, baked goods, sewing, clay sculpture, photography, and anything that could even loosely be called a craft, in the fair's competitions - sometimes winning. The girls taught themselves to swim in tiny, warm tide pools, and learned how to catch the illusive Dungeness crab of the Pacific Northwest. There was berry and cherry picking, resulting in kitchen smells so grand that every kid on the beach was attracted in a steady stream.

The cabin's greatest gift to us was time. Time for me to be a full-time Mom. Time to bake, cook, hug, kiss, hear and see. If the world fell apart, we wouldn't have known until we returned to Seattle.

Despite all the fun, Shari was still the outsider looking in on a world where she desperately wanted to belong, but didn't. Children made fun of her - her lisp, her stutter, her eyes. We often brought her school friends along with us to the beach, and that helped. But her melancholy never left her.

In 1971 I gave up my large modeling agency and became an events coordinator. Because my job required me to work long hours, I tried to include the girls in my business activities whenever possible. They helped with set-up and take-down; they folded, stapled, packaged, and arranged flowers. The sense of responsibility and accomplishment that the girls gained was invaluable, especially for Shari. Shari was successful at so much at a very young age while working with me, but times remained tough at school.

Shari was failing everything. Her kindergarten teacher, who knew Shawn, was quick to point out that Shawn learned everything quickly, so Shari should go home and ask her for help. When in the mainstream class, first grade was even worse than kindergarten. A new lunch pail, clothes and snappy hair bows could not help her read, do math, or spell. Shari was in tears every night after school.

The one good thing that did happen to Shari in the first grade was Toni Schlosser, Shari's special education instructor. Toni provided us with the one shred of hope to which we clung to for many years. I continually asked her if she felt Shari would survive. Her answer was always the same, "Yes, she will." Whenever I was discouraged, I would replay her words over and over in my mind.

Then came the big day. We were called in for a parent- teacher conference. This was a special one, not the kind the rest of the parents confronted. We dressed up, thinking it might help. We were faced with stern looks from the teacher and principle along with a table full of test results and graphs. We were told that Shari was not learning even the simplest tasks and that, if we were lucky, she might reach the fifth or sixth grade comprehension level as an adult. With even more luck, she might be able to learn a trade. They suggested that we put her in with those of "her own kind." To me "her own kind" meant blonds with dimples, people who can memorize every word on a Disney record-book set including the beeps telling when to turn the pages, people who loved God and believed on scruffy little knees in the joy of those beliefs, people whose kindness and generosity was unmatched. It wasn't clear to me what the school officials meant by "her own kind."

They suggested that I send my child to a school for the retarded. I could tell that they were uncomfortable having Shari in their "regular" classrooms. Inside I still felt like a child who had been summoned to the principal's office. I was not inclined to argue with them, but I asked them if they would agree to keep Shari in class for another year or so to see if things improved. They agreed. At that time they could have legally refused my request. It was not until 1975 that a law was passed requiring school boards to offer handicapped children an appropriate education.

This conference was also the first time I heard the word dyslexia applied to Shari. The multitude of tests that had been administered to her indicated that this was her problem. At that time dyslexia was a word which had a long history in the medical field, but was just being used in the education profession. At first people were so eager to have a name for a learning disability that it often was used incorrectly by educators as a catch-all phrase to describe any and all learning disabilities. I didn't know what it meant, but it sounded like a terrible disease. For Shari's sake, I tried to hide my fears. I tried to encourage her by telling her that having dyslexia was not a bad thing at all, it just meant that she learned a little differently. Shari was not impressed. She put her hands over her ears and said she never wanted to hear that dirty word again.

As I went through the education process with Shari, her life began to answer questions I had about mine. Similarities between my childhood and hers surfaced. Shari's report cards mirrored mine with comments like, "If she would only pay attention;" She lacks concentration;" "She is too easily distracted." I had been known as "Queen of Extra Credit" because I just couldn't succeed with the regular tests and reading materials. I began to realize why writing a check was so hard and why I can't read instructions for an appliance. I had never taken the time to think about why I memorized speeches or ad-libbed in my seminars and shows. When you can't read your notes on stage, it's the only alternative. Shari was a reflection of me in everything that she did. She was a reflection of my past, but she also reflected all the things that I couldn't provide for her. I was a learning disabled mom helping my learning disabled kid try to do homework. I felt more and more inadequate.

In 1975 Roger and I got divorced. I felt that I had failed miserably, and that, combined with my learning disabilities, contributed to my fear of being alone following the divorce. Less than a year later I married the first man I dated after our divorce, knowing the potential problems but choosing to ignore them. His children needed me; he needed me. Our marriage was a turbulent one in which we had to deal with the tragic loss of my step-daughter (which Shari describes in detail later in the book) and some serious health problems. I almost didn't make it through that time in my life, and at the time, I didn't care. Life had become too hard, ugly, and complicated. The knowledge that I was my children's only source of stability and the thought of what they were going through encouraged me to get well and stay alive. My marriage, however, did not fare as well. It fell apart at the seams after two years.

Through each mistake I made, I realized that my children had suffered, and this hurt me deeply. I don't know if I will ever come to terms with that. Maybe no parent ever does. All I know is that Shari was the one who was most devastated by each bump, each turn that our lives took. When Roger and I got divorced, she thought it was her fault because she was failing at school. I was unhappy, and Shari felt she needed to make me feel better because, in her mind, she was to blame. When I remarried, Shari went along with it trying to make the best of it; she wanted to smooth out the rough spots and be a perfect kid. None of the problems we encountered were her fault, but she always saw it that way.

At a very early age Shari was incredibly sensitive to others and to how they were feeling. She often felt responsible for things that had nothing to do with her, simply because she was so caring. When you are that sensitive, you read each face, each remark, each situation and wonder, "What did I do wrong? If I did this or that could I make everything better?" I believe that every remark, every frustrating situation, told her that she was not good enough the way she was. She searched until she found what she thought life wanted from her, and that was a good report card. Bed-making, dish-washing, even singing (which she began doing at age five), never earned her a star. Relatives and friends found it easy to make the comments that they mistakenly thought did not hurt her feelings. Out of fear for her safety and self esteem, I held her back from activities that she could have done because I was afraid for her. So many mistakes were made. Somehow, she remained resilient.

When Shari was in seventh grade, while I was in the midst of a marriage that was falling apart, Shari tried to reconcile the situation. She felt she needed a good report card to make herself worthwhile and to make the family proud of her, so she began learning how to learn. With nothing else to hold on to and our lives in complete shambles, she sat at the kitchen table every night and pushed the information into her head until it stuck. I was working. I was not there to stand over her and push her to do this. It was her choice. She found another way.

When she brought home her first 4.0 report card, I can only say that I was speechless. But they continued to come one after another. She maintained the 4.0 through the second divorce and a number of new schools.

Why? Because life wouldn't accept her any other way. She forced herself to fit where they said she never would make it. Did I support her? Yes. Did I understand her drive? Yes. She feared the world as much as I did. It was an unspoken feeling between the two of us. But she also saw me struggle. She saw me believe that my values and my chance at survival depended on someone else, and she didn't want that for her life.

Through eighth grade, ninth grade, and on through high school, our lives continued to change. I got married again, we moved into new homes, but her grades were always there like a trophy saying "I am somebody!"

I often looked at her and cried. She pushed herself so hard that, at times, I thought she would break. I wanted to stop her but she wanted to succeed so badly that I could only step back and watch.

Shari and I used to mark the days of school off on a calendar like a jail sentence. I used to tell her to just get through high school, that is all I asked of her. People said she wouldn't go beyond the fifth or sixth grade. People said she would be fortunate if she learned a trade. I cried at night wondering about her future, sad that I didn't have the money or the knowledge to fix her problems. She not only graduated from high school, she was fourth in her class. Currently my daughter is a graduate of the University of Washington and is going on to graduate school.

How does that happen? Is there some formula that you must follow? Love, the foundation of love is what does it. Admitting that you made a mistake, that you were wrong, gives your children permission to do the same. Even when your child is angry, you hold them close and tell them that you love them. Even when their pain is so immense that you are small in its presence, you say I will do everything in my power to help you through this. You let them know that no matter how bad it seems today, tomorrow is a new day and they can always start again. No matter how far away they go, they can always come home. Teach them to be responsible, capable human beings. Show them how to handle life so that when you aren't there, they can stand alone. Hold on to them with all your might through every storm so they know they are not alone. If you do these things, it won't matter that your child has learning disabilities or a handicap. For you have given them a foundation on which to stand that will hold them up through all of the blows that life directs at them.

Shari went through some very sad moments. A couple of times I thought she would lose her mind because she worked so hard. I mean literally working so hard that she couldn't push anymore. As I said earlier, she is resilient. I am convinced that all children are. Our mistakes as parents and teachers will only last if the mistakes are continually repeated. If we regroup, apologize, and try again, our children will forgive, and they too will learn that life's only real imperfection is making a mistake and not trying again.

We are given these precious gifts, children. We are as frail as they are sometimes, but children can often see far beyond our frailties. To them we are mom, to them we are dad, or teacher, or protector. We are the ones with all the answers, the ones with the great and powerful hand that can create what they need on a moment's notice. It does sound like we could never measure up to what they see in us, but we can. I didn't have all the answers, but I tried. I didn't make Shari into what she is today, but she is a reflection of me. A mirror image of what is good in me. Saying I am proud of her doesn't begin to express how I feel about Shari and all she has accomplished. Not because she went beyond the dreams that I or anyone else had for her, but because she dared to try.

Lynda Pressey

STUMBLING BLOCKS TO STEPPING STONES

CHAPTER 3

Before I was tested and found to have learning disabilities, I knew that there was something extremely different about me. From the earliest moment when I started to compare myself to those around me, I realized that I was not like the other kids in my neighborhood, or those in my classes, or even like my sister.

It was clear to me even at the ages of four, five and six that I heard, saw, acted, and even moved differently from other people.

Even when I got glasses, my eyesight was still bad in ways that I couldn't fully explain. Even if I had the ability to turn up the sounds around me, I couldn't seem to hear things clearly. Even when I was alone, I was distracted by noises and movements that no one else seemed to notice. Even when I tried to focus all the bottled-up energy that was inside me, I never felt that I was in complete control. Even if I stared at the page of my easy-reader book for hours, I could not make the words stop moving and jumping across the page.

Imagine being a little kid and having the world overwhelm you to such a degree that you begin to wonder if you are crazy, stupid, or retarded. Sometimes, I had to ask myself, what is wrong with me? Why am I so confused and mixed up? Why do I feel so out-of-order? Why can't I hear or see things like other people can? Since nobody knew exactly what was wrong with me, I just believed that I was strange, different, and dumb.

FILTERING SYSTEM

To a person with learning disabilities, a simple thing like shopping can be a bewildering experience. The lights, colors, and people are overwhelming. I didn't see each individual thing, I saw it all. I didn't hear one thing, I heard it all. I couldn't put order or priority to things; it was all a big, bright, noisy jumble.

I can remember my mom always holding my hand - someone was always holding my hand. If they hadn't, I would have always been lost. If something looked interesting, I would just stop and stare at it until someone realized I was gone. I was not frightened of things, I did not sense danger. I couldn't seem to think ahead, everything was in the here and now. All the pretty colors, the rushing people, everything was going and moving. It was as if the continuous movement around me invaded my brain with no pattern, control, or order.

One day, a local band of Hari Krishna were banging drums and dancing around on a Seattle street corner. I was waiting with my mom and sister to cross the street. The light turned and everyone started to move - except me. My mom and sister looked back to see me standing mesmerized by the flying pony tails and beating drums of the Hari Krishna band.

I would have stayed there until they packed up their drums if my mom hadn't collected me first. That's how I was! I would get sidetracked so easily - if something moved in a pattern and was bright and colorful, I would get caught up into it. Any previous thoughts were replaced by new thoughts, or distractions, in a matter of seconds.

A small attention span is a trait common to most children, but for me, it was a moment by moment occurrence. All kids stop and stare; all kids get caught up in rhythm and lights, but for me it was all-consuming. I couldn't remember things or think with commotion around me.

It felt as though there was limited space in my brain for information. I could only retain so much, and what I did retain was seldom matters of importance. Instead, it was all randomly selected pieces of information jumbled together in a manner that didn't make any sense. While other people could decipher the world's commotion, taking only the pieces of information that they wanted, I could not. My brain couldn't filter out the one noise I wanted to hear, like my mother's voice calling for me from across the street. Her voice became jumbled with the sounds of traffic, dogs barking, children playing. That was true with all of my senses. I felt bombarded and couldn't seem to separate what was necessary from what was not. In recent years, I have given a rather unscientific, but appropriate, name to the ability to control incoming sensory messages. I call it "The Filter System," and I do not believe that I was born with one, or at least one that works correctly.

This system allows you to sort out one object in a room filled with a hundred things, or listen to one conversation in a room where twenty people are talking at once. My audio (hearing) and visual (seeing) senses were not able to filter and segregate the stimuli around me.

Think of the affect a faulty filter system has on an individual. It affects concentration, conversation, and retention of what one sees and hears - how can you remember what you saw or heard when you saw and heard everything? It is a tiring state because I can't block out the unnecessary movements and commotion in favor of those that I need to experience. By the end of the day, I have used up all my energy in working to push the extra stimuli out and I feel exhausted and fatigued.

Having my senses overloaded all the time made me feel out of sorts and out of control as a child. It also explains why I felt like I was in the wrong place all the time (a lot of the time I was!). Directions were muddled with other pieces of information. Instead of remembering what my mother told me to do or where I was supposed to go, I would instead remember only pieces of what she said; and it was never the important pieces. I ended up being in the wrong place, doing the wrong thing, at the wrong time. The important information was replaced with the unimportant.

When I entered school, this problem became more pronounced. "Listen to me!" "Pay attention!" "Stop looking around!" "Stop talking!" "Why can't you remember anything I tell you?" "That isn't what I told you!" "Don't look out the window, look at me!" "Did you read any of the directions on your paper?" "Did you hear a word I said?" "Straighten up and look forward!" School added a whole new dimension to my life. At school I was not only a different kid, I was a bad kid.

Each distracting behavior displayed by students like me only serve to frustrate teachers and convince those who are unsure about our potential, that we are unteachable. The truth is that students like me can be taught to remind ourselves of what we are supposed to be doing and, if need be, isolate ourselves from the noise if our brains can't filter the noise out for itself. If kids are not taught to monitor themselves and their behavior, and that it's possible for them to take control of their behavior, it is likely that they will be the ones constantly in the wrong place, doing the wrong things, just about all the time.

As a child, I wanted so desperately to turn off the noise in my head, to calm myself down, to get control of my body and mind. But my control would only last for ten minutes and then I would be chattering, misunderstanding and running into things again. It wasn't until second and third grade that I received any help with my filtering system problems.

HYPERACTIVITY

When I was little, I was filled with so much energy that it was overwhelming. I didn't need a nap; I didn't need rest time at all. I had energy from morning to night. I didn't walk, I ran. When I was sitting still, my knee bounced or my hand patted the desk or table to some unknown rhythm in my head. I didn't have control of this energy; it had control of me.

I wanted to slow down because I was always getting into trouble with my constant movement. I knocked over glasses, tripped over things, ran into objects, moved too fast, talked too fast. Having glasses helped me to see and stopped some of my tripping, falling and habitual accidents, but it couldn't eliminate them completely for I was not only hyperactive but also had definite motor coordination problems.

I can remember the many times that I was just an accident waiting to happen. I would be filled to the brim with energy and ready to let it all go. My mom would sense the build up, and she

31

knew that either I had to clear my system or something would get broken or I would get hurt.

I don't know how this came about or who thought of it, but when I was having one of those energy filled days and I just couldn't hold it in any longer, I would take a pillow and lie on the living room floor. I would put my head on it and yell. I would punch the pillow and roll it in a ball. Then, I would put my head on the pillow and run around it sideways, keeping my weight on my head. That's how much energy I had. That's how badly I needed to get it out.

It was like a therapy session when I was finished with the pillow. I felt relieved and more in control. Once I had all the excess energy out, I would comb my hair, put my pillow away and go on with the day like nothing happened. It worked. My knees bounced less, my fingers stopped tapping and my movements slowed down.

When I went to sleep at night, I curled up in a ball with my knee's underneath me and rocked back and forth until I fell asleep. I couldn't lie still, not even if I was very tired. I had to rock, back and forth. I had to have at least one part of my body moving at all times or I felt an overload. This movement at bedtime helped me to calm down by releasing some energy so I could fall asleep.

I also rocked when I watched television. I didn't even know I was doing it. I would be sitting, watching TV and I would start rocking back and forth to some rhythm in my head. It was as if the rocking calmed me down and I could focus solely on the television program. If someone said, "Sit still and watch," I don't know if I could do it.

The rocking and movement continued for many years. In fifth grade we had to give oral book reports in front of the class. I went to the front of the class - which is a very frightening experience when you are self-conscious - and without even realizing it, I began to rock. I was telling the class about my book and within minutes I began my side-to-side rocking motion.

The other students would imitate me sometimes by speaking in a monotone voice, which I often tended to do. I was so busy trying to remember the facts about my book that I did not put any inflection in my voice. As they droned out the facts of some book, they would rock from side to side. Once they had made their point, they broke out laughing. I dreaded book reports that year.

Imagine what it is like to have too much energy. When you are an adult it means that you get more done in a day and everyone praises you for it. When you are a child, it means that you get in trouble a lot. How many times does the average kid hear "settle down," "be quiet," "stop that," "don't do that?" Now think of how many times a hyperactive child is told these same things. It is one thing to have the energy of a child and another thing to be hyperactive. When you are hyperactive, you are basically out of control and often behave inappropriately.

My mom was told to put me on a medication called Ritalin. It was being handed out like candy at the time. Every child that had a slight behavior problem was put on this type of medication. But my mom refused to put me on any medication, and I am grateful. I know that there are some children who can't get by without medication; it really helps to calm them. I also know of children that show no change while on drugs and others who experience minor to serious side effects. My mom felt, as I do now, that the use of medications was not the solution for me. She feared that it would just lead to further complications. Nobody could give her any concrete answers or projections for my future if I was to take Ritalin, they could only write out the prescription. That was not enough for her.

When my mother first told me about Ritalin, I began reading and listening to anything and everything that I could about it, as well as other forms of treatment for hyperactive children. Today, my main concern is that children with emotional and behavioral problems should not be put on medication only to keep them in control. The student's hyperactive behavior might be masked by the medication while keeping the child under control in the classroom, but the drug may also mask other problems that the child is having which need to be treated.

According to Jane Allen of the Citizens Commissions on Human Rights, there are documented cases of young people who experience such severe withdrawal symptoms when being taken off the drug Ritalin that they commit suicide. Although these cases are extreme, it should be of concern to all parents and children who use Ritalin and other drugs. These medications should not be handed out as a convenience or for a quick solution. It is a drug put in the same Schedule II category as cocaine, morphine, and opium by the Drug Enforcement Administration. This is a frightening fact. We must find other possible solutions. To me, any use of medication to control so called behavior problems should be given serious consideration.

There have been many studies done and clinics established for treatment of children with food allergies and other related allergies and intolerances. I know, because I learned at age eighteen that the reason I had so many ear, nose, throat, hyperactivity and respiratory problems was because I was highly allergic to milk, soybeans and wheat, and had slight reactions to chicken, peanuts and eggs. The foods I have just named are common food allergens, but people can be allergic to almost anything. Special testing facilities and clinics can diagnose these and other allergies that may influence behavior. These allergies can be controlled through diet, allergy shots, and other treatments.

Finding out about my food allergies changed my life. I dropped twenty-five pounds and was free from sinus headaches and stomach aches for the first time in many years. I found myself able to concentrate better because I felt better. I can only imagine what this allergy diagnosis could have done for me at age five or six. I may be the extreme, but I know of many children and their parents who have found relief from many ailments by a change of diet. It is worth looking into the treatment of food and other allergies as part of a program to get help. I know that there are many doctors who say that food is not a contributing factor with hyperactivity or learning disabilities. I also have heard other doctors say that these elements do affect one's abilities. For some children, it might not cause the problem but it might aggravate it. Whatever the case, I think it is important to check all the possibilities through the proper channels before resorting to medication.

I, like many children, had problems in several areas. There was no one cure for any of the ailments, yet it was important to separate one problem from the other. Whether you are a teacher or parent, before you act rashly, make sure that you are treating the right problem. Hyperactivity may be only part of several problems. Maybe that child is acting out and using his energy in destructive or distracting ways because he is learning disabled and can't function at home and at school as other children can.

Some people think that being in control is the most important goal that a child can achieve. As long as that student is in a resource room or calmed by medication, then the problem has been eliminated. A child will get passed along as long as she can keep quiet and not cause any problems. But what has she learned? Only how to hide and stay out of trouble? Covering a problem does not mean it is cured. We must look at the whole child. Separate, if possible, one problem from another and use the proper measures to treat that individual.

SMALL MOTOR SKILLS

Since my sister was two years older than I, she was in school before I was. She would come home from class with papers and projects. I really didn't know what school was all about, so Shawn would tell me about it and show me things that she had learned.

I remember one night my sister and I were sitting at the table with paper and pencils. On this particular night, she was going to try to teach me how to write my name. I took the piece of paper and a pencil and tried to follow each instruction. She showed me what finger the pencil should sit on, and I tried to hold it, but it felt uncomfortable. I held my pen or pencil on my third finger rather than my second finger from my thumb. From that first experience of holding a pencil, until I was eighteen years old, I never held my pencil on the correct finger.

That night, I learned each letter of my name and tried to write them. I tried to hold the pencil tight enough, but I couldn't. It felt awkward and uncomfortable. I kept pressing down on the paper to try to get control over the pencil and the lead would break. I would try not to press so hard but by the second letter of my last name the lead was pressing down on the paper again. My fingers felt thick and uncoordinated. My hand wavered and I couldn't keep my letters inside the lines. My writing was slanted and jagged, and the letters were all different sizes.

I was known all through school for my heavy writing. I pushed hard on the lead making my letters dark, sometimes even pressing right through the paper. I couldn't stay within the lines, I slanted my writing up the side of a page. I couldn't get my writing to be straight. It was like my hand was out of my control and would slant no matter how much I tried not to let it.

I learned to hate writing because my hand would hurt. The more I tried, the more it hurt. Writing was just one of the many tasks requiring use of my small motor skills that I found hard to do. Everything from threading a needle, to using a pencil, to snapping my fingers, to tying my shoes was hard for me. The smaller the skill, the harder it was. I felt as though I could not control the small little muscles in my hands. It was as if the sense of touch in my hand was not sensitive enough.

The skills that required small movements were hard because I tended to overdo. My hyperactivity caused me to use too much energy for most tasks anyway, but in addition I thought that by pressing hard and moving fast I would have more control. When I moved slowly or deliberately, I couldn't keep my muscles from shaking. Overdoing wasn't the perfect answer because, in the process, I made a lot of mistakes. But using too much energy, was the only way I knew how to react to my environment.

My eye problems combined with my coordination problems to make this lack of control of my small motor skills even more frustrating. I could see the hole in the top of the needle, my hand would hold the small piece of thread and then it would begin to shake. My eyes couldn't tell my hand where to put the thread and my hand couldn't coordinate itself to hold that tiny piece of string and put it through the eye.

Sally L. Smith, author of the book, No Easy Answers, the Learning Disabled Child at Home and at School, said that learning disabled children feel like they have gloves on when they try to do things that require their small motor skills. I agree. I felt like the senses in my fingers were muffled. That, combined with my lack of eye coordination, made the simple things of life seem impossible.

35

LARGE MOTOR SKILLS

Most behaviors don't involve just one of your senses. To write, I use my eyes as well as the sensory and motor skills in my hand. To run, I use my feet and legs, and my arms and my eyes guide my progress. Sometimes, I use all my senses together - that's when it gets even more confusing.

Having audio, visual, and motor disabilities, means that each part of my senses are affected in some way. Alone, each one of my senses has trouble, but I can handle it. Combining my senses in an activity means total confusion.

You need to understand this when I tell you about how I learned to ride a bike. Riding a bike requires that you use your large motor skills in all parts of your body and coordinate them to go forward, to turn, and to avoid crashing into things. It also requires hand, eye, and foot coordination. You must be able to coordinate what you see and hear with what you're doing with your feet and hands. Remember when I told you about going shopping and feeling overwhelmed by the sight, sounds and movement? Riding a bike is just another example and another form of how my senses would overload and be unable to function.

One year my sister got a little purple bike. It had a plastic basket attached to the front and a banana seat. My mom had managed to keep me on a "Big Wheel" up to that point. She figured that since a "Big Wheel" was plastic and low to the ground, there was probably only so much damage I could do to myself or anyone else. I soon graduated to a tricycle, but I looked at my sister's purple, two wheeled bike with awe. When Shawn grew out of that bike, I inherited it. I didn't care that it was a hand-me-down, I wanted that bike. Industrial strength training wheels were put on and away I went.

Time passed and I was getting impatient with the training wheels. I asked my parents if they would take them off. They came up with a whole bunch of reasons why it couldn't be done, and dad found a lot of other projects to do around the house But finally they could put it off no longer. The training wheels came off, and with determination I got back on the bike thinking, how hard can it be?

I had plenty of energy to move the pedals and steer the handle bars - that wasn't the problem. The problem was putting it all together. When I was riding, everything seemed to happen too fast. My reaction time was slow and once I realized the space between the house and our stone retaining wall was too small for me and the bike to fit through, it was too late. I had already hit the house.

I had a lot of trouble determining space and distance. My eyes could not accurately determine how far, how wide, or how deep something was.

SPACE, DISTANCE, REACTION TIME

It became common for me to misjudge the size of a curb and either overstep it or under-step it. Either way, it was frustrating because everywhere you go, there are curbs and steps and things to walk over and around.

I had my glasses on. I could see, but it felt like my eyes would deceive me. Everything was out of proportion to me. I fell down, around and over things. Some people can see the stairs that they're about to go down before they reach them. They see them out of the corner of their eye with their peripheral vision. I know that I have peripheral vision, but it isn't very good. I don't see the flight of stairs unless I look down. I have to look directly at every step and every curb or I will trip or fall.

Some people can judge the height that they need to step in order to maneuver at a curb while they're walking. Although I'm better at this as an adult, as a child, each thing I did had a process. I couldn't blend everything. I didn't automatically know what size step to take while walking up stairs. My senses seemed to be separated, each needing calculation time before they could work together. How high is the step? How high do I lift my foot? Just taking a simple step requires many different processes to work together accurately. If they don't work succinctly, you fall. And I did many times.

Our house sat on a steep hill on a road that none of the kids in our neighborhood were allowed to ride our bikes on. Fortunately, we had a sidewalk that went all the way around our house so that I could ride in circles. The path was very narrow and it was easy to run into things. In the backyard, there was a playhouse in one corner and a picnic table in another. On one side of the house there were steel poles in cement put there by the previous owner. They were my major obstacle because the path was so narrow and there was also a large stone retaining wall on one side. When I came to the front of the house, I had to dodge the two cars that were parked high on the hill of the driveway and bypass the garbage cans. Then came a small sidewalk in front which passed by a concrete bordered flower bed. When I came to the end of that sidewalk, I had to make a sharp turn to the other side of the house. If I didn't make the turn, I landed in the neighbors' yard, which I did on occasion. There was also a sidewalk on this side of the house, so it was smooth sailing until I got to the end and had to make another sharp turn or land in a tall, leafy tree. If I made the turn, I was in the backyard again dodging the picnic table, playhouse, and sandbox.

Since I can describe this path, it is obvious that I traveled it a lot. I walked it, ran it, and even rollerskated it, but nothing compared to riding a bike around it. I would get the pedals and the front wheel going to make the turns, my eyes would watch the scenery go by, and my mind was trying to take it all in. The one thing I couldn't seem to combine with all of this going on around me was, "How do you stop that bike?" Remember my reaction time is slow, I misjudge distance, and now something is coming at me that is going to hurt me if I hit it!

My mom got used to hearing a crash in the backyard. Like everything else that happened with me, she learned to prioritize. She learned not to make a big deal out of my crashing on my bike because it happened so often.

When a baby falls down and everyone makes a fuss about it, the baby starts to cry. Have you ever seen that before? The baby doesn't cry until she sees the reaction of those around her. Had my mom made a big deal about crashing on my bike or all the other things that went wrong in my life, I probably would have been even more nervous. Instead my mom believed in me and encouraged me, so I would get back on the bike and try again. If she had made me feel helpless, I don't think I ever would have learned how to ride.

I later discovered that when she heard a crash in the backyard, she'd say to herself, "Oh, Shari is riding her bike again." When other people came over to our house and heard the crash, they would say, "Oh my gosh, what is that?" My mom would say rather casually, "Oh, Shari doesn't know how to stop her bike, so she just hits the playhouse."

On a daily basis, my mom would find me in the backyard crying after I hit any number of things that were in my way. She would put antiseptic on my cuts and scratches. She'd pick me and my bike up and say, "Well, try it again." I had the resilience of a Tommy-Tippy cup. I would go down for the count, but I would always come back up again, as long as my mom believed I could do it. I could have had a concussion, but I'd get back up on that bike and try it again.

I recently received the transcripts from a PBS television program, Bodywatch, regarding people with learning disabilities and/or dyslexia. During the program, James Duke, Jr., M.D., and Albert Galaburda, M.D., associate professor of Neurology at Harvard Medical School, talked about the new research being done on the brains of dyslexic people. They are now finding that there truly is a circuiting problem, among other things, that can be detected and is probably the source of the short circuiting or malfunctioning of our brains. I used to laugh and say my brain short circuited and that's why, under pressure, I would run into things on my bike or would be unable to draw forth even the most familiar information from my brain. Now I know I was correct in my thinking.

SENSORY NERVE ENDINGS

Recently I was watching one of the national talk show programs whose topic was autism. With the movie <u>Rainman,</u> which is about a man who is autistic, there has been a sudden influx of information on the topic of autism and autistic savants (those who have special talents). Physicians are now finding out more about these people and the type of world that they live in.

On this particular program, there was a woman who, with years of help and therapy, was able to come out of her world of autism and deal with life as a normal, functioning person. I found her story fascinating. The most interesting part was when she talked about her symptoms.

The talk show host asked her why the autistic person doesn't want to be touched, why they react so adversely to loud noises and tend to close themselves off from human contact and the world which surrounds them. Her answer was that her nervous system would get overloaded, her senses would get more stimulus from the touch of a hand or the scratch of a lace collar on a blouse than a normal person would experience. She said that this extra stimulation from a touch was not just uncomfortable, it was excruciating; that a loud noise is not just loud to an autistic person, it is deafening. Although I certainly couldn't relate to all that this autistic woman had gone through, listening to her made me feel that in my own way I could understand the feelings that she described about sensory overload.

When I was little, I remember hating to be tickled. And when you're little, everyone wants to tickle you. At first, I thought it was funny, but then it would turn into what only can be described as a feeling of pain. It's like hitting your funny bone. For some reason you laugh, but at the same time it hurts.

I was the most ticklish kid I've ever known. Every nerve in my body was set off when I was tickled. My skin actually hurt to the point that if you didn't stop tickling me, I would cry.

My skin felt itchy and crawly all the time. Certain fabrics would bother me more than others, but no matter what type of fabric it was, I constantly felt like there was a bug crawling on me. I would look and nothing was there. I would scratch, but the itch was never satisfied.

I liked being hugged and cuddled, but jostling and wrestling was not the best way to handle me. First, because I was hyperactive, wrestling with me only got me more rambunctious. Second, all that sensory stimulation would overload me and I would want to withdraw; the stimulation was too much.

I also remember not liking to have anything touch my skin in repetition. I recall sitting in church with my Grandma and Grandpa. Grandma was lovingly holding my hand. She rubbed the top of my hand with her thumb while she was listening to the sermon. The pain was terrible. I'm talking about actual pain from a soft, repetitive caress. More than three light touches and I couldn't stand it. I was afraid to take my Grandma's hand off mine because I loved her and didn't want to offend her. So I kept her hand there, but it hurt. Sheets, clothes, the glasses on my nose, a light caress - just as my senses were overwhelmed with noises and movement, my skin was overwhelmed with touch. I felt everything ten times more than the average child.

With all of this over stimulus to my senses, it is no wonder that I found it hard to sit still or get comfortable. I remember sleeping with my Grandma when we got to stay at her house. My sister would fall peacefully asleep when she slept with Grandma. I on the other hand would wiggle, squirm, and drive my Grandma crazy trying to get to sleep. My skin felt the new sheets and the nightgown that my Grandma had for me when we came over and I wasn't used to the fabric. New school clothes, freshly washed blue jeans touching my skin, or a scratchy slip to a party dress were unbearable for me.

I know that in some ways I must have made people a little crazy and uncomfortable. It made me feel crazy and uncomfortable, too. No matter where I was, I saw too much, felt too much, and heard too much. In reality I guess my whole body, even my skin, was without a filter system. Without this filter system, I experienced sensory overload every minute of everyday.

Just as the autistic woman described, I, too, found noises abrasive and disruptive, even at levels that other people would consider acceptable. I didn't like big noises, unexpected noises, and noises that were erratic. When I say erratic, I mean music that didn't go in a pattern that I could follow. Conversations and TV shows with changing volume levels bothered me. Guns and bombs on the TV bothered me. I liked music that was repetitious, and silence was better than noises that I couldn't control. Loud noises to me were in some way painful. I didn't have the necessary filter system that I needed to monitor or control the noise, so instead, I had to remove myself from it physically by leaving the room or covering my ears.

I didn't like noise, let alone loud noise; but at the same time I found myself unable to distinguish words clearly unless they were loud, near to me, and even more important had something visual to help cue the meaning. If I was looking directly at the TV, I understood what was being said. It was almost like I was lip reading. I combined the visual with the auditory for understanding. But if you moved me away from the TV and gave me only the auditory to connect with, I often misinterpreted and literally couldn't understand what was being said. The words were muffled, fuzzy, and jumbled together. The same thing happened in the classroom. If I was given directions without the teacher looking directly at me, I didn't understand what was being said. The teacher had to look at me, make sure that I was concentrating on her, and speak in a very slow distinct way. When the teacher did this, I understood and followed her directions.

Music is a little different. Even though it really doesn't have a picture to associate with it, it can be played over and over again until I learn the words. Also, although it may not be visual, it has a beat and a rhythm which helps me to understand and follow it better than just words alone. For that reason, I can keep music at reasonable levels.

It is a standing joke between my husband and me that if I am home, the TV is turned up so loud that the neighbors can tell what show I am watching. It is also a joke in our house that I always answer a question with, "What?" I learned to respond this way in school even if I heard what someone asked me because I needed to turn around, face the person speaking to me, and watch them as they said it to me again. I needed to hear the question twice to reinforce and clarify what those words were. Saying "what" meant that they would say it again, and implied only that you didn't hear it, not that you couldn't understand it. I learned very early not to trust my ears or my eyes. Both of them deceived me and garbled information. Saying, "what" was just one of my many shields to cover what I could not do.

From my earliest memories bright lights, bright colors, horns honking, crowds of all sizes, noises of all kinds, have bothered me. As a child, I learned early on to survive by isolating myself in silence. I enjoyed being alone because that was my filter; that is how I dealt with the sensory overload. I preferred dim lighting to bright lighting, a firm touch to a soft caress, no noise to any noise, repetition and patterns to not having a pattern, soft colors to bright colors, and being alone rather than being in a group. I didn't realize just how different I was from other kids my age until I got into school and I could not control the atmosphere. When I was at home, I could isolate myself, I could control the amount of noise, light and movement. At school, I had absolutely no control. My differences became more pronounced in a busy room full of children.

41

I have read that children with learning disabilities are said to have an immature nervous system. I believe in this theory whole-heartedly. It's not that this state is permanent, but for a few years they will be the itchy, ticklish, distracted, and overwhelmed students who sit in classrooms everywhere. It will take time for them to catch up. It will take time for their nervous systems to mature so that they can calm down. I still feel itchy and ticklish, and my knee still bounces to that unknown rhythm in my head. My nervous system may not have completely matured, but it did get better with help, time, and determination.

STUMBLING BLOCKS TO STEPPING STONES

CHAPTER
4

When I was still very young, my mother went back to work. With my dad's encouragement, she opened a modeling agency in the Seattle area. The agency grew and Mom taught classes and trained models for fashion shows and other modeling work.

When I was about three and my sister was five, we would go to the agency and watch my mom. We usually went on Saturdays when my sister wasn't in school. Shawn took some of the children's classes with the other kids who were enrolled, and although I could have been included, I managed to get myself in enough trouble that pretty soon my mom was wondering why she had brought me.

My sister could sit quietly and listen or participate in the classes. Even though I did not have bad intentions, my hyperactivity would soon get the best of me. I would run around making people laugh with my crazy antics. I would try to sit still; but the more people laughed, the funnier I got. The kids in my mom's classes were there to learn, yet I was running around like the class clown, talking a mile a minute and loving all the attention. My mom tried to be patient, but there was only so much that she could take.

I recall one Saturday morning I woke up early and I ran into my mom's room, ready to wake her up so she could take me to class. When I jumped on the bed, only my dad was there. Then I ran to my sister's bedroom and jumped on her bed, but she was gone, too. I started running around the house to see where they were hiding. I looked outside to the driveway and the station wagon was gone. I started crying when I realized that they slipped out while I was still asleep.

I cried over the fact that they had left me, and I cried even harder when I realized that I would end up going with my dad and his friends to Denny's for breakfast. They would sit around talking and I'd be bored. Then we would come home and I'd play by myself for awhile, or maybe we would go to the hardware store - Dad's thing to do on a Saturday.

Oh, how I wished I could be with my mom and sister. After realizing that I had been left behind, I had a long talk with myself. "Now, Shari, you're gonna be good. Next time you go to class you are going to be so good that Mom will keep taking you." I'd tell myself all of the things that I was going to do and how great I was going to be, how I'd sit nicely and quietly. I had it all planned out by the time they came home from their day of classes.

When the following Saturday came, I made sure that I got up in time to beg my mom to let me join her. I gave a good argument, "Mom, this time I'm going to be sooooo good. Really Mom, I mean it! You won't even know that I'm there!" She was not completely convinced, but she gave in. I held true to my promise for about five minutes and then I was off and running again. It just wasn't in my nature to sit still. I was allowed to go to the agency every now and then, but never as often as Shawn.

MRS. SAGER

Since my mom was working full time, she looked for a baby-sitter and housekeeper. Many baby-sitters had come and gone in our house. Few knew what to do with me, and since I was the one who was home most often, we would definitely need someone who was very patient.

My mom put an ad in the paper, asking for a grandmotherly type to take care of two small children and do household chores. The ad was answered by a woman named Mrs. Sager - and Mrs. Sager got the job. I would still have to go to Denny's with my dad on Saturday when my mom didn't let me come to class, but during the week I had a friend, a baby-sitter, a lunch-maker, and a story-reader in Mrs. Sager.

She was quiet as she walked around the house making lunch and doing the laundry, and I always had to look really hard to find her. The only sounds she ever made when she wasn't talking were when she would hum church hymns. She talked quietly, walked quietly, and was reserved but loving. For a child like me who made noise everywhere she went, this lady was shockingly different.

Mrs. Sager read stories to me at least once a day. I only had a few books, so I listened to my favorite stories over and over again. When she read to me, everything was very precise, and she pronounced everything perfectly. I didn't know how to read at all when she first came to our house, but even after I did learn how to read in school, I still preferred to have things read to me. I learned very early on that I understood things better when I heard them than when I read them.

Days with Mrs. Sager included stories, a nap (so she thought), watching TV, listening to Disney records, and playing with my toys. Mrs. Sager's stories were good, but her food was even better. She made the best fried chicken and mashed potatoes that I ever had. Sometimes she would make up a big chicken dinner and have it waiting when everyone came home from work and school. Now one would think that I would take advantage of her ability to make such good food, but at lunch I opted for one of two things. I liked Campbell's Tomato Soup or Pork and Beans. Nothing homemade, just pork and beans right out of the can was fine. I ate so many beans that she would call me the "Pork and Beans Kid." And the butter sandwiches that came with my beans were the best. Just enough butter and just enough bread. I loved her so much that she could have served me anything and I would have eaten it.

The best days were when she let me eat in front of the TV. Those were special days, my napkin under my chin and my beans on a placemat on the floor. There I sat with my lunch watching, "I Dream of Jeannie" or "Bewitched." When lunch was over I had to take my nap, but as long as I got to eat lunch on the floor watching TV, I didn't care.

The days with Mrs. Sager were the best. She really loved me and took good care of me. For the time that she was with us, we were very blessed. She had a profound effect on my life. When I was sick or upset, she was always there. She never yelled at me or even scolded me. She had a way about her. All she had to do was say "no," and I would do what she said.

I was a different kid than most, but she never made me feel that way. I respected her and she respected me. I was little, but I remember how she talked to me, always with a calm voice reminding me of what to do and telling me what was happening. I never felt confused or out of sorts around her. She looked at me when she spoke to me and it helped me to follow what she was asking me or telling me to do. She calmed me somehow, and it made our time together peaceful and easy.

I didn't know until I was older, but my mom and Mrs. Sager talked about me and the fact that I was not only sick a lot, but I was just plain different. She told my mom that no matter what anyone else said, I was going to make it. She was right.

She knew that I was going to make it and she treated me accordingly. She was everything good, and life was better because of her.

She was a religious woman, and the reassuring presence she had around our house reflected her deep faith. She seldom talked to me about God, but there was something about her that made me understand more about God than any Sunday School class I ever attended. She didn't have very much; her life had been very difficult, but she went to church every Sunday and lived her life the best way she knew how. I learned from her. She was an example to me in the way that she treated me, the way she cared about my family; and the way that she acted and reacted helped me understand God. I know that I was in her prayers. Even though she is no longer alive, I have blessed her name in a prayer every night since she first became my friend.

DISNEY RECORDS, COMMERCIALS, AND JINGLES

We used to have our record player down in our family room. I would sit on the two steps that led to the family room and listen to my Disney records for hours until I could recite whole albums word for word and song by song.

I had Peter Pan, Robin Hood, Brer Rabbit, Aristocats,

Country Bear Jamboree and others. My mom would come down and sit next to me on the stairs and sing the songs with me. We would follow along with the pictures in the book that came with the records. I couldn't read when I first got these records so I would just listen for the "beep, beep, turn the page." The funny thing was that I would memorize the record and include the "beep, beep, turn the page," as if it were part of the dialogue!

As I look back on those Disney records and the time I spent memorizing them, it occurs to me that even when I was little, I had the ability to memorize things if I heard them in repetition. But more than repetition, if information was set to music, if there was a pattern or rhythm to follow, I would learn very quickly, and I would remember them for a long time.

Words are just words to me, they always have been. I have to hear someone say something many times before I can remember it or even understand it. The written word is even harder, I have to read a text book chapter up to ten times before the information has any meaning. The more difficult the information, the longer it takes me to learn and the harder it is to remember.

But, something happens when you take the written or spoken word and add to it in some way. Although at times distracting, pictures in a book help me to make an association with what the words are trying to convey. While watching a movie, I can hear information and associate it with a picture and that works even better for me. If I put the picture and the words together in repetition, and then add a little beat or music, I can learn just about anything.

I don't know why this is, and I don't know if all learning disabled people learn this way. But for me, I need to bombard my system with the information before it will make sense. Hearing works the best, but all of my senses need to receive the information in repetition before I will truly understand it.

One of the most effective teaching forms that I have ever experienced as a learning disabled person, appeared as a series of educational spots broadcast on Saturday morning between cartoons. The series was called "School House Rock." I learned everything from how a bill becomes a law, to the Preamble of the Constitution. Through music and animation, I learned about pronouns, conjunctions, adverbs, times tables, and so on. They played different programs every Saturday and then once they had all been shown, they would repeat the broadcast.

These short programs gave me an opportunity to use my audio skills, memorization skills, and my ability to associate information with pictures for recall. I would watch these programs over and over again, until I could sing all the words to the songs. The songs had a pattern that helped me to memorize. The pictures gave me something to associate with the words I heard. They showed the programs in repetition so I could learn them, and the characters and songs were interesting which made learning much more enjoyable.

When I eventually became frustrated with not being able to learn in the way I was being taught in school, I basically had to go back to the things that had worked for me   when I was younger. Going back to my childhood made me realize that I have always been smart, but I didn't learn in a traditional way. I had to go back to the Disney records and "School House Rock" format of teaching with sight, sound, pictures, and repetition all put together before I could start to learn in a way that worked for me.

PRESCHOOL

Before I went to school I thought I was different; when I did go to school, I knew I was different. When I started preschool, I thought it would be so fun. What is preschool anyway? Just finger-painting and other activities designed for kids to learn to play with other children. I learned right away that I didn't fit in.

My teacher was probably a very nice women, unfortunately I never saw that side of her. I think it is safe to say that I drove her crazy. She wanted all of her students to sit down and be quiet; a feat that is next to impossible with preschoolers. I was hyperactive, had a lisp, and wore thick glasses with a patch over one eye. I was easily distracted, my attention span was about as short as it could be, and she thought that I was going to sit still and be quiet. Not likely.

Mrs. Sager could get me to sit still and be quiet. She didn't use harsh words and punishment, she simply kept things quiet in the house, read me stories, and reminded me what I was supposed to be doing when I got off track. She believed in me and I was happy and successful when she was around. When I began preschool, I was always being told to sit down, be quiet, get in line, don't touch that, pay attention, and so on. There were all these rules and I always seemed to break them. I was one among many now. The teacher had many kids to look after. I was either getting lost in the shuffle, or getting in trouble.

Because my mom worked, she sometimes couldn't pick me up right after preschool. Often, I had to stay after school with the teacher until my mother arrived. My teacher lived above the classroom; she had converted her basement into a preschool. On the days when my mom picked me up late, my teacher and I would walk up the flight of stairs that led to her home.

It was an ominous flight of stairs because during the day if you even looked at that stairway, you would get in trouble. It was off limits to all students. I remember some of the little boys in the class putting their feet on one of the stairs when the teacher wasn't looking and feeling like they were really pulling something off.

After climbing the stairs with my teacher after school, I sat in a stiff-backed chair in the teacher's living room and waited, hoping my mom would get there soon. Sitting in my teacher's house made me realize that she was a person and that she had a life, pictures of her family covered the walls. I wanted to tell her that I had a life, too. A life in which I was a totally different kid than the one she saw at school. I wanted to tell her that I was a normal kid most of the time, in fact I was even a good kid most of the time. I was in preschool then. I had the simple thoughts and wishes of a of a preschooler. But my feelings were very real. I wanted to explain myself to her, but I could tell that I made my teacher very uncomfortable. When the two of us got upstairs, she would leave the room and I would sit in my chair and not move. I didn't watch TV and the radio wasn't on; I just sat in her living room alone.

RIDICULE

I remember one day in preschool when we were all sitting in our chairs facing the front of the class. The kid sitting next to me was hitting me and calling me names. I think the standard phrase at the time was that I had a mouth full of polluted underwear - now there is a frightening image! When I went to tell the teacher, she was standing at her desk and gathering some papers for her lesson. I told her what happened and she said, "I'll handle it, now go sit down." I went to sit down and the same kid who had made the underwear comment had turned my chair under the desk. All the chairs had been facing forward, but now mine was facing backwards. I turned around to sit down in a hurry. I fell on the floor and my head hit the back of the chair; the whole class was laughing. My dress was up in the air, and I was trying to figure out how I didn't see that the chair was turned around. I must have looked like a real stooge, the perfect one to ridicule.

So there I was on the floor crying, the kids were laughing, and I was saying, "Mths. Coats, make em thstop that." When the teacher picked me up off the floor and put my chair like the others, I thought she was really going to go after the menace sitting next to me. But instead she said, "Now Billy, I don't think we should do that anymore." Somehow this wasn't exactly the reprimand I had in mind for Billy. For the rest of the year, I learned of the great creativity that children have when making up names to call other people. I learned to fight back. I also learned that fighting back usually got me in trouble, not the ones who tormented me.

PATCHES AND PERMANENCE

When I was four I got thick glasses and thought they were awful. I felt ugly and the glasses reinforced my feelings that I was different and stupid. At almost the same time, I was also given a plastic patch to wear over my good eye so that my bad eye would have to work harder. I thought this was the worst. I knew there was a reason for the glasses and for the patch; but when you feel ugly, those reasons don't seem to matter. The glasses, the patch, and my lisp combined to make me stand out in class. Now I also had differences that people could see.

The only friend I had that understood me was a kid named Ricky Peele. He was out of school for a while because he had been in an accident and had injured his eye. When he came back to school he was wearing a patch similar to mine. He probably hated wearing a patch about as much as I did, but I was glad someone else knew what I was feeling.

I thought that both of us having patches would bring us closer together. So, I tried to befriend him. I brought him get well cards, told him that I hoped his eye would be better soon and that I understood how it felt to wear a patch. We became friends, and one day I even went over to his house to play after school. As long as the patch was on, we had something in common.

Although both of us wore patches, his was only temporary. One day I came to school and his patch was gone. We were no longer friends after that. With his patch removed the permanence of my problems was reinforced. He only had to be different for a little while.

I hated my patch and my glasses even more after his was removed, and from that point on, I started asking for contact lenses. I was four years old, in preschool, and asking for contact lenses. I thought if I had them I would have lots of friends. I kept asking and the doctors kept saying no. I wore my patch for over a year and I was growing more and more impatient, until somehow my glasses and patch mysteriously disappeared out of the back of our station wagon. "Gee, Mom, I don't know how that happened!" Even at four I didn't want to be different and would go to any extreme to fit in.

When I went in to be refitted for new eye-wear, the doctor said that my eyes had improved considerably. I wouldn't have to wear the patch anymore! I was thrilled - yes, thrilled - until they gave me a new pair of glasses that were just as thick as the first pair. And I thought they had broken the mold when they made my first pair!

NOAH'S ARK

When I was little, my sister and I didn't share a room. We each had our own place with our own things. I loved my room, my dolls, my records, and my bunk beds. I enjoyed going into my room and arranging things and reorganizing where my dolls would sit on their shelf and in what order my toys should go into my toy box.

At four and five, my family was the most important thing to me. The outside world didn't understand me, but at home I felt loved. My mom's love for me made me feel secure. Each thing that she gave me was a prized possession. I wouldn't clean out my room and give things away because each Christmas gift or birthday gift was so precious.

During the summer before my preschool year, one of the local gas station chains had a promotion. When you filled up your car with gas, you could collect a Noah's ark; and with each subsequent stop you could get a pair of animals. Each week was a new type of animal. We had to buy a lot of gas to get all of the animals, but it was worth it. I had every animal that Noah had, or at least all the animals that the gas station thought Noah had.

I loved that ark. It became my favorite toy. I took it with me wherever I went. That one toy could keep me busy for hours. There were about thirty pairs of animals and I continually found new ways to walk them up the plank and into the ark.

One day, I decided to take my ark to school for show and tell. During playtime, some kids came over to see my ark but I wouldn't let anyone touch it. Later, as I was putting each of the pairs of animals away, I noticed that one of my turtles was gone. I searched the floor, the table, anywhere that it could have been overlooked; but it was nowhere to be found.

I was so upset that I didn't know what to do. The teacher told me to put the ark away, but I wouldn't. I had to look through all the pairs of animals to see if I had missed that turtle somewhere. Finally after a few minutes passed she came over to my desk and firmly said, "Put that away." I told her what had happened, but she didn't seem to understand how important this was to me. She just said in a louder voice, "Sit down and put the ark away!"

She could make me sit down but she couldn't make me stop thinking about the missing turtle. Remember, I don't have a filter system. I should also add that outside noises, movement and color can make it difficult, if not impossible, for me to concentrate, but even more important is that worry or fear was like a noise in my head, to the point that I couldn't function or concentrate until it was relieved. If I was upset about even the smallest of things, I couldn't concentrate.

My brain didn't seem to have the capacity to put things aside when I was told to do so. Whatever feeling I was experiencing, whatever worry crossed my mind (whether it was about today or tomorrow), was in the present. And these worries were not even rational, they could be worries or fears about something that would never happen, but the anxiety was there. The feelings tended to circle around in my head almost like a broken record. At four, at fourteen, and even now I notice that the record still plays. My protection from it is greater now but I still have trouble concentrating if I am worried about anything.

I think the reason why I worry in the first place is because my brain is so out of order that I forget, misplace, and misunderstand things. When I was younger, I was sure that if something went wrong, it was my fault. After all, if your brain doesn't work so well, how do you know that it wasn't your fault? Even when something didn't go wrong, I assumed that it was just a matter of time before it would and that I might as well start worrying now. It was painful because I could never get away from this emotion.

I heard the teacher saying, "Sit down!" But all I could think about was my turtle.

When I saw that nobody understood my grief over the lost turtle, I took things a step further. I can't believe at four years old I had the guts to go against a rule just to find a turtle, but I did. I walked out the door of my classroom, and up the driveway looking carefully for the lost turtle. I was gone only a few minutes when I heard my name being called. I just had time to turn around when the teacher grabbed me by the arm with a grip that was very tight. I was dragged down the hill with the teacher yelling at me all the way.

When we got into the room, I was taken to a chair and put in it. I didn't sit, I was put in it. It was in the darkest corner of the room and I was not allowed to participate with the class in any activity for the rest of the day. I sat in the dark and was told to think about what I had done until my mother came to get me. I know the teacher was upset about my leaving the class, but if she had listened to me in the first place, it wouldn't have happened.

As illustrated by this example, it is very easy to get angry with children like me. They ask more questions than any other kid, they talk out of turn, they distract themselves and those around them, and generally can be very difficult to keep up with and understand. Their patterns, rituals and actions make sense to them, but not to those who surround them. Sometimes they become out of control and can't seem to stop doing whatever it is that disrupts their classes or makes it hard for others to concentrate.

That is why you have to repeat things over and over again for us. What we are doing, where we are going, any hint of change, any new material or rule must be explained time and time again so that the learning disabled child has time to adjust. And if we express fear or worry, you need to listen and help us find a way to cope, or remedy the situation by showing them that there is nothing to worry about or that you will help them find what they are looking for.

The things that were precious to me, like a special gift from my parents (the ark), weren't part of my teacher's world. She couldn't understand why I got so out of control over seemingly small things. In her eyes, I was a strange little trouble maker, wandering around the room looking for a turtle. When she didn't understand me, it just exaggerated my fears and worries, that day and every other day that I spent in her class.

If my mom had been at school when I lost my turtle, she would have helped me look for it. If we couldn't find it, she would have convinced me that somehow it could be replaced. That's all you have to do. My mom knew how my mind would fret over things until they were resolved. She would calm me by finding a solution.

When my mom came to pick me up that day, the teacher and she had a conference. When their conference was over, my mom came to the back of the room where I was sitting with my head down on the desk. She took my hand and we left the room. When we got in the car she had me explain my side of the story, then she told me the teacher's side of the story and how dangerous it was for me to go out in the driveway without an adult. We talked about it until I started to feel better and I understood why I had gotten into trouble. That was it. My mom didn't have to punish me; I was hard enough on myself as it was. She just explained the situation to me, assured me that we could get another turtle and I felt better.

I didn't seem to get angry at other people for not understanding me as much as I got angry at myself for being so different and doing things so strangely. As a child, I wanted my brain to turn off, but it wouldn't. It was like that missing turtle was a missing piece of me, a piece out of order that wouldn't be settled until I found it. Losing things, noise, a fight with someone I loved, a change in a schedule, and any number of minor things unsettled me to the point that I couldn't function. These are things that I felt from the beginning. There was always a missing turtle, always something to worry about.

ALTERNATIVES FOR PRAISE

My mom could just look at my sister and find many things to praise. Shawn achieved high grades, had good manners, followed directions, and did all the things a good little girl is supposed to do. My talents were not that obvious. My mom had to look for things that I was good at and had to teach me things so that she would have something that she could praise me for.

When you have challenges, like learning disabilities, you can imagine the creativity that went into finding things that I could successfully do. The truth is kids love to help. Kids like to be included and to be given responsibility. My mom looked at the situation this way: if you praise a kid for making her bed, she will probably make it more often. If you say, "Why is this room such a pig sty?" it will probably remain a pig sty. If you clean the room for your kids until they are twelve and then ask them to start doing it, you have missed the boat.

I could have been a messy, disorganized person. Instead, I became the neatest, most organized person in our household simply because I was asked to help and to take on responsibility - and then was praised for it. I hear kids say, "Mom, can I help?", "Mom, can I mix the cake?", or "Can I turn on the dish washer?" Why not? Show them how to do it, watch them as they learn, and when they can handle it on their own, you won't have to do it. In the back of your mind, you're thinking parent-like thoughts: "What if they mess up?" Did you ever mess up? Did you learn from it? Especially with a learning disabled child, you need to give them extra time to learn the task, and more grace time for mistakes. Praise them and the grace time will be even less.

My mom couldn't praise me for conventional accomplishments, so she taught me things around the house - everything from making my own lunch, washing dishes, washing clothes, putting rollers in my hair, hemming my own pants, mending holes in my socks, to vacuuming and dusting. These were things that nobody else wanted to do; but if she kept praising me, I thought it was great. It wasn't what I was doing that was important, it was the praise that came from doing it. My mom didn't gush all over me about sweeping the floor, but she noticed it and praised me for doing the job well.

My mother was doing more than just finding things to praise me for, she was making me self-sufficient. I have met learning disabled people who can't take care of themselves. They don't have the basic skills to make it on their own. It is a crime for anyone, no matter what their challenges, to be forced to depend on other people. My mom made sure that if something should happen to her that I would be able to take care of myself. In turn, I received praise and responsibilities which other people seldom gave me.

As time passed, it went beyond just cleaning and doing household chores. Cleaning became my way of organizing myself and my brain. I know it sounds funny, but it is true. Being in a noisy, disorganized environment made my brain even more disorganized than it already was. At school, I had no control over my environment, but when I came home I could organize and reorganize my room and somehow it made me feel more at peace and more in control.

Once I learned the skills of cleaning and organization, I developed patterns and order around these skills and how they should be done throughout the day. I was only four or five years old, but I had a rigid pattern for the day all worked out. Each task had an order and a place. I would make my bed, get dressed, wash my face, brush my teeth and so on. I learned not to deviate from that order. With order in my day, things went faster and smoother. The older I got, the more I relied on a pattern and became used to it. If that pattern was interrupted, it took me twice as long to accomplish the task. Ask anyone with learning disabilities, and they will tell you the same thing. If they have problems like mine, they will agree that the only way to keep up in this life is to be twice as organized and prepared as the next person. Once you learn a routine, you stick to it.

MAKING THE BED

Once you get into a routine for your day, it is hard to break. It makes it uncomfortable to sleep over at other people's houses because it disrupts your daily agenda. Because it takes so long for a learning disabled person to cope with changes, it is no wonder that we fear them so much and prefer to stay with a rigid, even boring, pattern over things that are new. Our brains work so strangely it is better to have sameness than to disrupt the pattern.

When I learned to organize myself and my environment, this out of control feeling decreased. I found that I may not be able to have control over all the changes that might occur in a day, but organizing my things and space was a way to be prepared when a change came about. When you are organized, there are fewer surprises. Since my brain wasn't organized, I just learned to organize everything around me to compensate.

When my mom taught me how to make a bed, I loved it more than anything else. You start out with a mess and when you're finished, there is a nicely made bed. There is a beginning, middle, and end to the project, and the finished product would always bring me praise from my mom. I became good at bed making - as good as I could possibly be, that is.

Bed making was the first part of my morning routine and I always wanted it to be right. If I didn't do it right the first time, I would take it apart and put it back together again. This is an important point, for when you learn these routines and rituals, you also feel the need to make it perfect. What starts out as simple organization turns into a ritual; your brain feels uncomfortable unless the pattern is not only completed, but performed perfectly. You will keep doing the ritual or pattern to the point that it is annoying because it calms your brain and makes you feel in control.

After I made the perfect bed, I would then pile all of my stuffed animals on top and arrange them in a different way every day. Then I would call my mom in and show her my magnificent bed, and she would tell me how great I was.

One night, my sister and I were going to have a slumber party in her bed. I thought this was very exciting because I was still at the stage where I had bunk beds with a Peter Pan spread. My sister had a double, four-poster, French Provincial bed from Sears, and I was going to get to sleep in it!

At three o'clock in the morning, my sister got up to go to the bathroom. When she came back into the bedroom, she started screaming at the top of her lungs that they just better get that crazy kid out of her room.

As I said, I was set in my routine. When she got up to go to the bathroom, I thought it was morning. By the time she got back, I had already made the bed!

DON'T GIVE UP

When my mom sold her agency and opened a production company, she started doing shows and productions at shopping malls. During her shows, the mall became our second home and we were there whenever we weren't in school. I learned about the business this way, running errands up and down the mall, carrying ribbon and signs for the booths, and working backstage at the fashion shows. I learned to be around people and how to speak to adults and to shake hands. These are social graces that were taught through experience. In school I was a fragile little kid; at a show I was shaking hands and talking to mall management with ease.

Over the last seven years of public speaking, I have met many kids who are like me. In school, their peers and the school system itself may label and pigeon-hole them into a certain group. Outside of school, it's different. They might be an outsider at school, but at the same time be the leader of their 4-H group, or the head cashier at the store where they work. I hope that these kids will hang onto their successes and not give up. Because I knew there were other things that I was good at, I didn't give up. In school I was considered a resource room kid; at the mall I was needed and could do anything they wanted me to do. All someone had to do was show me how.

My mom's shows always drew large crowds. I watched from the sidelines and saw how my mom put things together. I knew that my mom had one year of college, a few night classes and the rest was sheer determination. I watched her in amazement, how does she do it? It made me want to do better. I wanted to be more in control, to be able to think on my feet. I wanted to be successful. I would stand in the crowds, push my glasses up on my nose, and wonder when it was all going to come together for me.

Whether I was at the mall, the modeling agency, or running errands with my mom, I was included. Sometimes I got in trouble because I was too loud or not acting appropriately, but I was included. My mom had me with her because she wanted to protect me from the world; she thought if I was with her, I would be safe. Maybe in my heart I knew she was protecting me, maybe I wanted her to protect me. Protected or not, I learned a tremendous amount from these experiences. In many ways those experiences were my education.

SINGING

In her search to find things that I was good at, my mom looked at her own childhood experience as a performer. She was a singer and dancer from the age of three, so it seems appropriate that when I was five years old, she asked me if I could sing and proceeded to teach me everything she knew. I was so young at the time I didn't really know if I could, but from that time forward I was a singer.

Through her business connections, I had the opportunity to sing in public before I even realized I should be scared. Anytime that it was appropriate, I would put on my little costume, walk out on stage and sing. I wasn't afraid, not even nervous really; I loved it. From the first time I sang, I was in tune and I have always been capable of learning songs quickly. For me, singing was equated with sweeping the floor or making the bed and getting praise for it. The applause was my praise. I would take off my glasses and be somebody else for that three minutes on stage.

I sang, "Somewhere Over the Rainbow," "Ma, He's Making Eyes at Me," and "I Didn't Know the Gun Was Loaded," which was my favorite because it was about a woman named Miss Effie who goes around shooting people just for the fun of it, and then says, "I didn't know the gun was loaded!" By accident, she shoots the sheriff in the hip and then tries to get out of it by snuggling up to the judge. During this part, I would do a Mae West impersonation. Here was this little kid doing Mae West; the crowd would go wild. By the end of the tune, the sheriff's wife shoots Miss Effie, and then gives the same excuse as Miss Effie always had, "I didn't know the gun was loaded!" I would sing the last "I didn't know the gun was loaded!" then I'd yell, "yee-ha," shoot my cap gun in the air, and run off the stage. Lisp or no lisp, I was a hit.

Had it not been for my mom's productions, I may not have had the opportunity to perform. If my mom had not asked me if I could sing, I might not ever have tried. I was so fortunate that my mom pulled my talent out of me early and found things that I could do well. Being able to perform made me feel good about myself at a time that was so crucial. At school I was the weird, unteachable kid; easily ignored. And at the same time I was performing and gaining praise at home and on the stage. It kept me balanced and positive amid the tough times.

FOREVER BOXES

My mom felt as any mother would towards her children. She did everything she could to ensure our safety and well being. I know that when she looked at Shawn, she felt security. Shawn has always been so intelligent and mature. But what about Shari? My mom has expressed to me so many times the fears that she had about my future. She would lay awake at night wondering who would take care of me if she wasn't there. She taught me to be self-sufficient by teaching me basic skills and responsibility around the house. But would that be enough?

She understood me better than anyone else. There were family members who had wondered about me, family friends who unintentionally or intentionally made me feel like an outcast; she had reason to be concerned. Even if my father took care of us when she was gone, how would he deal with this child that required so much extra care?

My mom had only one sister, who died of cancer when I was no more than three or four. I know that when my aunt died, my mom became even more intent on making sure that we were taken care of. If she went on a trip, she would buy an insurance policy at the airport and have it sent to us. (That's something she still does.) At Christmas and birthdays my sister and I always received a gift that wasn't a toy. My sister and I each had a small TV, a sewing machine, and other appliances by the age of twelve.

She made sure that we would literally never have to depend on someone for money if she died. She put the insurance in our names so that there would be no contesting it. Some people don't like to think of death because they are afraid it might happen. My mom saw death as reality. We did have my dad, but she wanted to leave us with tight security that would insure our college education and living expenses if something happened to him as well.

My mom feared not being there for us in the future and I feared losing her, too. A life without my mother would have been so

59

different. She always included me and was there for me. I'm sure that all kids go through a phase where they have fears like mine, but for me there were so many reasons why the fears persisted.

Again, it goes back to a routine and a pattern. I was so afraid of a disruption, the outside world was scary and home was safe. The thought of losing my parents meant losing that safety and protection.

In my own funny way, I created an insurance policy for myself. It had no monetary value, it wouldn't have been worth anything to anyone but me. I could not insure that my family would never die, but it gave me this little bit of security knowing that I had a piece of all of them to hold onto.

There was a television show on at Christmas called the "Littlest Angel." It was about a little boy who was called up to Heaven by God. When he was called, he left in such a hurry that he left behind his most prized possession, a box filled with all of the treasures that he found on his travels.

When the little boy reached Heaven he became the littlest angel, but he was not happy. He missed his treasure chest so much that he began to create a great commotion. Seeing how upset he was, God let the littlest angel go back to earth and get his precious box.

When I saw this show, I decided that just like the littlest angel, I too was going to find a special box and keep all of my treasures in it.

The box that I found was made of tarnished gold metal on the outside, and purple velvet lined its interior. I don't know where I found it, but it became a safety deposit box of sorts. It held the trinkets that only a child would cherish. The napkins from my lunch bag that were never used because they held a special drawing or message from my mom, dime store dolls, and treasures that I found on my adventures.

It held all of these things, but more importantly, it held something that belonged to each one of my family members. My dad's broken watch and a black comb from his medicine cabinet. I took some little dolls of my sister's that she no longer played with, and when Shawn got her hair cut, I collected some of her hair and put it in my box. From my mom, I took an earring that didn't have a mate, and fabric from a dress that she made for herself. If my family cast things aside, I found it and put it in my box. Little did they know I was cleaning up behind them, treating these little pieces as if they were gold. Those pieces would be there if my family wasn't. When my dad smoked and I feared losing him, I would look through my box fingering each of his items. When my mom was sick and overworked, I would go in my room and look through the box. When my sister went to school all day and

I was at home and missed her, I would take that funny tarnished little box and look through it again. The box was filled with my family; it was my security, my forever box.

THE SHOELESS BRAIDER

The memories that I have from kindergarten are not those of finger painting and nap time. Although I remember those things and a few of my friends, it was during my kindergarten year that I realized I could not learn like the other kids.

The only detail of this year that sticks out in my mind was when my teacher handed back our arithmetic papers, she inadvertently held my paper so that others in the class could see that I hadn't done very well. And, of course, the kids in the class made fun of me. Those kids would forget that paper and forget laughing at me. Even the teacher would forget the incident. But I couldn't forget it. I wanted to grab that paper out of her hand and run. I didn't. Instead, I just went home crying. After that incident, I had hives every day before I went to school.

That day, my mom and I made a trip to the drug store. We went to the corner drug store to the shelves where all the paper doll and coloring books were. Workbooks were on the bottom shelf. These workbooks were for reading and math. I became used to these trips; every time my papers came back to me at school we went to the drug store to get a workbook.

I guess my mom and I were hoping that it was only a matter of repetition for me to master the skills of reading and writing. We kept getting the workbooks, and I kept getting numbers and letters backwards. 3 was E, 5 was 2, and S was 2. B and D, F and E, L and I, any letters that looked alike at all I would use incorrectly, and just plain letters in general were backwards for me. The workbooks couldn't change the fact that I had dyslexia, and it was showing in just about everything that I was doing.

My mom would have helped with my homework, but she couldn't. She had learning disabilities, too. My dad could have helped, but he was working all the time. My teacher obviously didn't know what dyslexia was or I don't think she would have held up my papers in front of the class which embarrassed me.

My mother did the best that she could for me. Every time I came home from school in tears, she would teach me how to do something else, another song, another skill. She would get my mind off what I couldn't do and put it on what I had accomplished. Praise and more praise, always reinforcing me so that I wouldn't give up.

On one of the days I came home crying, instead of handing me a cookie or patting me on the head and saying, "It will get better," my mom got out three brightly colored ribbons. Each was about a yard long. She took the ribbon and tied them together at one end.

That day she taught me how to braid. I tied a knot at the end of the ribbons and then attached that knot to the back of a chair or the leg of a table, and braid for hours. Once I made the braid I would undo it and start over again. There was a pattern to it which made it a great activity. For a kid who was easily distracted, it was amazing how long this task kept my interest. I liked to see the colors go together. I enjoyed the hand pattern, and the visual pattern, and how the two combined together. I would start with three separate ribbons and end up with a piece of art when I was done.

I could look at a braid, but I didn't know how it was made. When I looked at things, they were just what they were. I couldn't take them apart and put them back together in my mind or guess their contents. Life was like a slight-of-hand trick. People see a normal kid and assume that they know how to do simple things. I didn't know how to do even the simplest of things until someone taught me. I'm sure people often wondered why I could belt out a song but couldn't snap my fingers. That is the gap that all learning disabled kids seem to face. They may be brilliant in a very difficult area and ignorant in the simple graces of life.

Braiding got me through kindergarten. I took my ribbons everywhere I went. The only time that I couldn't braid was when there was no place to tie my ribbon. One time I wanted to bring my ribbons in the car, but I didn't have anywhere to tie them. So my mom said sort of off-handedly, "Why don't you just tie them to your toe."

"Tie them to my toe? What do you mean, tie them to my toe?"

"Just what I said, take off your shoe and tie them to your toe." She said it, and I did it. Have ribbons, will travel. In the car, on the front porch, wherever I went so did the ribbons.

On one occasion, I brought the ribbons to school to make a big braid for show and tell. Granted, it would be an unusual show and tell, but it was better than nothing. During math time, the most dreaded part of my day, the ribbons began to burn a hole in my pocket. Everyone around me was counting and working hard on their 1+1's and 2+2's. I couldn't do what they could do, and I just kept thinking that if I could show them what I was good at, it would change how the teacher and my classmates thought of me. If I could just show them that I could braid, they would like me.

In the middle of math I showed everyone my talents. I pulled the ribbons out of my pocket, took my shoe and sock off and started braiding. The kids started to look at me; I think they were a little surprised at the sight. I thought they were looking at me in envy because I could braid, but it wasn't long before the teacher looked up and saw me without my shoe. That was it, my chance was ruined. She wasn't interested in the fact that I could braid, she just wanted me to get my shoe back on and to put the ribbons away.

No, braiding didn't change my life, nor did it make up for being behind in school. Neither could bed making or singing. But it was the small things that helped me through school until I could find a way to learn.

CHAPTER 5

When I entered first grade, it was with great anticipation. I couldn't have been happier to have completed preschool and kindergarten. The patch over my eye was gone and I felt like I was starting over again. I was looking at first grade as the "Big Time," and I thought that this year would be different. I kept thinking to myself, "Oh they just didn't have enough time to get to know me in my other classes. We only went half days in pre-school and kindergarten." I thought that if they had more hours with me, they would like me better. I guess my logic was a little off.

I don't know why I remained optimistic. It would seem that after two years of failure, I should have been beaten down, but I wasn't. Summer had renewed me. The time I spent with my mom and sister, and the little time I spent with my dad, was good. I was ready to try again.

Little children are so amazing. They have an enthusiasm for life that is unbridled. They get down but they don't stay that way. When I fell off my bike, my mom would just tell me to get back on, and I did. When I did badly in school, we would go get a workbook or she would teach me something that I could do around the house, and things didn't seem so bad. My mom handled all of my ups and downs in a matter-of-fact way, so it made me feel that my problems were not the end of the world.

When first grade started, I was glad to be in the building with the big kids. Kindergarten was in a separate building, but now I was in the same building as my sister. I also thought it was great that now there wouldn't be a nap time and we would go to school all day long. I can remember groaning about going to school as I got older, but in first grade it was a real privilege.

I went in on the first day filled with my usual energy. When I found a seat that looked good, I took it. Of course, I picked the front row. I wanted to be in the front row because that's where all the action was going to take place. As always, I liked to be right in the middle of everything.

All the energy that consumed me when I was standing up sent me running, not walking, everywhere; and it made me talk louder and faster. When I sat down, my energy went wherever it could: to my feet or hands, tapping, clicking, or stomping. It never occurred to me that I might be annoying someone. I was too busy making noise.

The first day of school was always very important. My mom put a note in my lunch and I wore my favorite new school outfit. On the first day of first grade, I happened to be wearing some very shiny, new Mary Jane patent leather shoes. I looked at them all the way to school as if they would go away if I didn't make sure that they were still there. When I sat down in my chair, class hadn't started yet so I began talking to the people around me. At some point, I started tapping my feet. My shoes sounded awfully good on the newly waxed floor. Just one tap, then two, then three, then both feet tapping to beat the band. The girl at the next desk started tapping her feet and then a little boy joined in, and then another. Pretty soon everyone in the class was tapping their feet and having a good time.

Then the teacher walked in. Everyone except me stopped tapping. I was so busy tapping, so caught up in my rhythm, that I didn't notice the teacher standing next to me. I felt a clunk of metal on my head. It wasn't a hard clunk, but a clunk all the same. It didn't hurt so much as it surprised me. I looked up to see the teacher standing over me. Her pen, which had just hit me in the head, was ready and waiting to strike me again.

She told me to stop. I got the message loud and clear and my feet stopped immediately. I looked at the teacher, then looked at my shoes, and the line from the Laurel and Hardy movies came to mind, "Look what you've gotten us into this time, Ollie!" The only problem was that I didn't have an accomplice to blame. It was just my shoes and me. The teacher's pen and I became very close that year.

I was so mad at myself. I had wanted to be good that day, to make a good impression on the teacher. Now here it was five minutes after the first bell and I was already in the hot seat.

That first day I got the first look of many from teachers that said, "Why don't you act like your sister?" My teacher knew my sister, so she certainly had someone to compare me with.

I had seen this look so many times before. When friends of the family came over for dinner, they would ask Shawn how school was going and would talk to her about all the wonderful things that she was doing. Then when they were through with her, they would turn to me. I usually didn't have much to say. I had the exaggerated view that when Shawn walked into the room everyone applauded. When I walked into the room, I usually tripped over something, skinned my knee, and spilled a drink all in one fell swoop. My entrances didn't offer much cause for clapping. I learned to hide out when company came.

I laugh about it now, but it was painful then. I rambled on about things that nobody was interested in, I talked out of turn, talked too fast, my speech was garbled at times, and in my zest to be included, I tended to speak loudly, and often interrupted people. Some of what I said and did didn't make any sense at all. My parents were used to it, the company was usually left puzzled by this strange kid. I could show them how I made a bed or how I could make three ribbons into a braid, but they didn't care about those things. No, they didn't have to say it out loud either; it appeared on their faces. They said it with their pressing looks and pressing questions. Sometimes they just ignored me. In time I came to appreciate being ignored. My mom didn't acknowledge that I was an outcast, but I knew it was true.

I learned that first day of school that my differences would not be tolerated. No tapping of shoes, no talking out of turn, nothing out of the ordinary would be put up with. "You will fit the mold here," is the message that I received. You see, my teacher's mold probably worked for most of the kids who walked through her door. Most kids could be alike without much effort. They could conform to the straight line that my teacher drew. I don't think that my teacher was a bad person, she just didn't allow room for any differences. Unfortunately, I was as different as they came. I would never fit her mold or walk her line. I made her uncomfortable with my fragmented thinking and my out of control movements. I was not a bad child, but I was looked at as such because she couldn't figure me out.

Imagine that frustration. I don't have any idea if she knew what was going on in my head. I don't know if she knew what dyslexia was, but she knew that she wasn't reaching me. The glasses wouldn't have scared her off, the lisp could be corrected, but what about the rest? In a class of many, what was she to do with me? Maybe it was because she couldn't find a way to get inside my brain and fix it that she so often made me feel inadequate. If she couldn't teach me, she had to label me as a bad kid; otherwise, she had to label herself as a bad teacher.

My teacher didn't know how to help me, so she sent me to a resource room. I don't remember when it happened, probably a few months into the year. I was tested again and again, and without notice I just started lining up at the door with some of the other kids from my reading group who were going to the resource room. I was scared as we walked down the big halls, but that fear went away once I met my new instructor, Mrs. Schlosser. She was tall and thin with a soft voice. I knew then that she was kind and would understand. She didn't move quickly or talk loudly, and didn't have bright posters hanging on the walls to distract me. Maybe the lights were softer there, or maybe it was just her presence that turned what might have been a bad experience into a good one.

I loved going to Mrs. Schlosser's room because she was so nice. It was quiet, and the quiet calmed me. I felt less nervous and more in control than I ever did in my regular class. In her room, I was safe. We worked on workbooks and listened to "Puff, the Magic Dragon" in the background, and I was with kids who were struggling like myself.

The thing that bothered me about going to the resource room

was leaving the classroom while the other kids stared. All our teacher would have had to do was to explain to the other kids in our class that we needed some extra help and we were going to see another teacher. Something, anything, would have been better than the silence. Kids are so curious. If you don't tell them what is going on, they will make up an explanation. From the first time that we lined up at the door and left our class, we were known as the "stupid kids."

Before I started going to school, my mom had instilled in me a wonderful sense of confidence. At this point in my education, I had not yet lost all of that. The funny thing is, when I was told to line up with the hyperactive, fidgeting, out of control kids going to the resource room, I looked at them and thought, "Oh, those poor kids." I felt sure that a mistake had been made when I was included in this group. I had no idea that I was just like them! It took only a little while before I realized the truth.

The stigma of separation that came with being a resource room student was more than just being misunderstood; it was realizing that from the first day that we stood at that door, we were not missed. The activities of the day went on without us. Not just the activities we struggled with, but activities we would have liked to do took place while we were away.

The lack of explanations to the other students in my regular class and to me about my challenges, combined with the fact that we missed out on the everyday activities with the other students, made the process of fitting in even more difficult. Even then, I felt that it was easier to get rid of us than to find a way to teach us and to create acceptance for us in our regular classroom.

A, B, C, D

The thing that I remember most vividly about first grade was our first lesson. We would all go to the back of the room and sit on the floor. My teacher would sit on a chair next to a big colored board with all the letters of the alphabet written on it. She would take a big pointer, point at each of the letters, and the class would say the letters out loud in unison.

I was eager to learn, and I ran to the back of the room so I could sit in front of the group. I would watch her point at the letters, but I didn't have any idea what they were. It seemed that no matter how many times we did this exercise, I just couldn't put meaning to the symbols. Everyone would say the letter and its sound out loud; I would just go along with what they said. My brain felt confused by all of this noise and I couldn't respond immediately. All the letters just jumbled together and looked alike.

I wanted to figure it out; I wanted to have the answer. But by the time I figured out which letter the teacher pointed to, it was usually too late to respond or everyone else had already said it aloud. I would hear them say it, look at the letter again and think, "Oh, yeah, that is a B." I heard them say it, I even went along with them and said it, too, but only later would the actual recognition would set in. Even when I got the letters right every now and then, I was very slow to learn the alphabet, letter by letter, and sound by sound. When I did learn the alphabet, I could only recite it if I sang it. I could not tell you which letter came before the other unless I sang my way through the whole alphabet tune to that point.

Yes, eventually I learned the alphabet. I would love to describe to you how I did it, but I'm not really sure. It was basically like everything else. It took much longer to make sense to me than it did for anyone else. The information could go in over and over again; I wouldn't understand it or put the meaning to that symbol until finally one day, if I kept working on it, it would start to make sense. I never stopped reversing letters, I could not always guarantee that I would recognize a letter correctly, but in time my recognition of letters and the sounds that accompanied those letters improved. Time was always the important element for me. I needed more time just to get the information into my head. The memorization and skill level for a task came later.

I started out sitting up front when we all did the exercise of learning letters. As time went on, the teacher started to call on people individually and I knew I didn't know enough to say it out loud. The teacher would call on me and all I could do was look at her and make a good guess. The harder she would look at me, the less I could think. The information was too fresh, it wouldn't come out that easily. I couldn't just look at a letter and have it figured out; I had to search my memory for the answer. It was in my head but always hidden. The teacher wanted the answer, but how could I tell her it was stuck?

That's what it felt like. It was stuck somewhere and it was just a matter of time before I could get it out. It was there and the teacher wanted it now. The pressure would build and finally I would just blurt something out hoping it was right. She would give me that "I'm disappointed in you" look and I'd sink into the floor. Before long, I stopped sitting up front and wasn't excited about going to school.

After learning the letters, we were supposed to learn how to read. It was no surprise that I ended up in the lowest reading group. The words were jumping all over the page and bouncing from one place to the next. There was only one line per page in those easy reader books and still the words danced!

Reading. Putting those sounds, those letters together to form a word was the most difficult thing I have ever had to do. Sitting in our little circle, the teacher would ask us to read out loud. I had a lisp which embarrassed me, and then in my embarrassment, I had to make sense of the black marks on the page. The letters moved and switched themselves around as if they were trying to trick me. The light in the classroom was too bright and distorted the words. The picture above the sentence distracted me and added to my frustration.

I used to pull the book close to my face thinking that the words would stop moving or that they would be more in control closer my face. I'd do anything to keep them still. But bookmarks, my finger and holding the book close to my face only worked for so long. I could probably hold the letters still for the first two words of a sentence, and then I was back to letters getting reversed, my eyes missing words, seeing words backwards or leaving words out of a sentence.

I wanted to blame it on the lights, they were just too bright. Then there was the noise that the other kids made; if they would be quiet, I could think. Then I thought, it's the pressure, if they weren't looking at me I could do it. I was learning disabled. That was my answer. I just didn't know what that meant at the time. And because I didn't know it, I constantly asked myself, "What is wrong with me?"

By the middle of the year, I learned to sit in the back of my mainstream classroom and hope that no one would call on me. I thought, "If I'm silent no one will see me, they will pass over me if I'm not too loud." I was a kid who wanted to learn but learned to hide in fear of being called on. I tried to fade away, but I was never quiet enough to disappear completely.

I never did learn how to read during my first grade year. I could stumble through an easy reader but I couldn't truly read and comprehend. I didn't have time to understand or remember what I was reading, I was too busy being frustrated, trying to keep the letters still, recognizing what the letters were, what sound went with the letter, putting the sounds together correctly to form the word and then putting the words together in a sentence that made sense. I could never understand the sayings, "reading for pleasure" or "leisure reading." There was nothing pleasurable or leisurely about reading to me.

LEADER OF THE PACK

On the playground or in the classroom, I was a misfit. I didn't feel like I was as good as the other kids around me; it was only when I was with the kids in my resource room, or with other kids who were different for some reason, that I felt comfortable.

70

If I was around kids whom I thought were better than I was (and that was most people), I felt like I owed them something. I learned early to make fun of myself or let them make fun of me, because I didn't know that I deserved anything different.

I was drawn to those who were like me, but more than that, to those who were worse off that I was. I was drawn to them because they made me feel that I was needed; without me, they just wouldn't make it. I wanted to be needed, to feel that I was taking care of someone. I couldn't fight for myself but I could fight for the others. Their pain was mine. The situations could be far removed from my own, but I could put myself in their shoes. I wanted to save them in the way that my mom saved me. I could include them in the same way that I wished to be included.

It started early. I became the leader of the misfits, and I planned to save them all. Anybody could be in my group as long as they smelled bad or picked their nose. If someone had problems which tended to exclude them from the mainstream they fit perfectly in my group. I would give pep talks and fill them full of my wisdom. I even brought a Bible to school one day. I couldn't read it, but I told my little misfit buddies that if they got down on their knees and prayed, everything was going to get better. I had a message to keep them all going, and their friendship and needs kept me going.

BILLY

Billy came to school everyday with his clothes dirty and worn out. He smelled so badly that most people didn't want to sit next to him, especially at lunch time. It was at lunch time that I used to sit and watch Billy eat. I was amazed at the sight. He got a school lunch through a program for disadvantaged kids and he'd eat the whole thing. He ate the spinach, the carrot and raisin salad, everything. The kids sitting around him would make fun because he ate even the worst parts of the lunch. And it was the way he ate it - he didn't even breathe, he just ate it fast until it was all gone.

When I was little, I thought of Billy as the kid who smelled badly, wore dirty, torn clothes and ate what the rest of us would throw away. Now I realize that Billy was an abused and neglected child. That school lunch was probably the only food he had all day. His clothes were dirty because no one washed them. He smelled because no one made sure that he was clean.

I was drawn to him because the teacher looked at him in the same way that she looked at me. She seemed frustrated with both of us. It seemed that Billy was always in trouble. On the playground or in the classroom, it was always Billy who was doing something

71

wrong. I often felt a sense of injustice on his behalf. I was so much like him, that I wanted to explain to everyone why he did what he did. Sometimes I even tried, nobody really listened though.

Yes, he was loud. He probably would have been considered a behavior problem. He smelled and kids made fun of him. Wouldn't you become a behavior problem, too? He was only in first grade. Couldn't someone have seen the neglect and helped him? He would defend himself against the taunting kids and the teacher would get mad at him. He was ignored because he didn't fit the mold, so he would cause a disruption and draw attention to himself. I was only six or seven and I knew what he was doing, getting attention in the only way he knew how. I had done the same thing myself. I used to watch Billy on the playground. Nobody played with him. I would see him chasing the girls or lifting up his shirt at them. The girls would urge him on and then tell the playground teacher what he had done. I started watching him and staying close by at recess. When I would see him start to lift up his shirt at the girls, I'd run over and say, "Billy, you know what is going to happen. You will lift up your shirt and the playground teacher will get mad." He'd look at me, look at the girls, and pull his shirt back down again.

Somehow Billy became my responsibility. He was my friend, so I could overlook the smell. He needed me, so the torn clothes and the fact that he would eat without breathing didn't bother me.

SARAH

Sarah was a little girl, probably the littlest girl in our class. She seemed frail and she always had a runny nose. Like me, she wore glasses. They were little and blue with a cat-eye shape. I was drawn to Sarah; she needed me. Somehow, I was her protector.

Sarah was smart, I think the teacher really liked her. It was the kids who picked on her, partially because of her size and partially because she was quiet. She was easily disturbed and that's what the bullies tended to look for. If they couldn't illicit a reaction, they would give up.

One day on my way home from school, I was walking to the crosswalk near our school and I saw Sarah crying. When I asked her what was wrong she pointed to the hill. I still didn't understand so I asked her to explain.

She said that everyday when she went home she had to walk up that huge hill. On the way up, all the boys who lived near her would taunt her and make her afraid. Every day it got worse, and today she was too afraid to walk up the hill.

I felt so sorry for her. Another little one that needed me, I thought. The mouse turned into a lion and I couldn't let her go up the hill by herself. On the other hand, I didn't want to go up the hill either. "Sarah, why don't you come to my house?" I said. Sarah was a little skeptical, but I convinced her that it was the best way to go.

When I got this brilliant idea, I didn't consider the fact that I lived about a forty-five minute walk away and she lived about fifteen minutes away and that we went in opposite directions. I didn't think about what my mom would do when I walked up to the door with a stray kid or what her mom would do when her child didn't show up from school. No, all I could think of was that I didn't want her to go up that hill and have to face the bullies.

I took Sarah home with me. We had a nice walk, she stopped crying and I talked like a tour guide telling her as much interesting information as I could think of about my neighborhood. When we arrived, my mom was waiting at the door for me. I said, "Hi, Mom. I brought a friend home with me." My mom didn't mind, it's just that she was wondering what my little friend's mother was doing.

We called Sarah's house and her mother came over in a rush. I think she was mad, but she didn't say too much. She just grabbed Sarah's hand and shuffled her into the car. My mom said my intent was right, but I couldn't just bring home stray children without telling anyone in advance.

"But Mom, she was scared to go up the hill!"

"Shari, no more stray kids, okay?"

"Okay, Mom," I agreed.

I didn't bring home any more stray kids after that - just stray animals.

GINNY

Ginny was about as wide as she was tall, and she wore every color and style of clothing in layers. She thought she looked great, everyone else thought she looked funny. Her hair was bright red, cut bluntly around her head, and could have looked nice if it was ever combed.

Like all my other misfit friends, Ginny became one of us. It was easy, she just fit right in. She reminded me of a story that was popular when I was growing up called, Pippi Longstocking. Pippi was a little girl who had to live alone when something happened to her parents. She had red hair that was done up in braids that stuck out from her head as if they were wired. She wore mismatched clothes, and she always had one sock up and one sock down. That story was Ginny's story. She obviously didn't have anyone at home showing her how to dress and nobody was combing her hair. In my eyes, she became Pippi.

The kids at school made fun of Ginny because she looked so

unusual. They called her "Fatso" during lunchtime and on the playground. The other students wouldn't sit with her. But I knew how badly it hurt. Billy smelled bad, Sarah was afraid, I couldn't learn and Ginny looked like her clothes came out of a garbage bag. We were all left out for different reasons but could relate to each other all the same.

I was the leader of this group, they were my wards. I looked after each one as if they were my children. Looking at them and feeling their pain made me forget my own. I wanted to protect Ginny most of all. There was something about her. I knew her the best of all of them and she became my closest friend during first grade.

Ginny was the first friend I invited to visit my family's beach cabin. Only my best friend could come to the cabin, my favorite place.

The first time that I invited Ginny to our cabin I got a little insight into her world. When we went to pick her up, my mom got out of the car to go meet her mother and let her know where we would be. Before my mother made it to the door, Ginny came out and met us on the sidewalk. My mom asked to see her mother but Ginny said that she wasn't home. Then my mom looked at her watch and said, "It's close to seven, she should have been home from work by now, right?" Ginny said, "Oh, sometimes my mom doesn't come home until real late."

Ginny assured my mom that it was okay for us to go, so my mom got back in the car while Ginny and I went in the house to get her suitcase. It seemed funny that she hadn't invited my mom or Shawn into the house with me, but when I saw the inside of the house, I knew why. There were dirty clothes everywhere. Dust was so thick you could write in it. There was on old tattered chair pointed directly at the TV set. Surrounding the chair were empty cereal, cracker, and cookie boxes.

Ginny later told me that her mom wouldn't come home until late at night or even early in the morning. Ginny was afraid to go to bed, so she would sit up all night watching TV and eating out of boxes until her mom came home. I started to understand her weight problem. She was neglected just like Billy.

The whole house was in a state of disarray and disrepair. It was hard to believe that someone lived there. Ginny's room was no different. It looked like a storm had blown through it. Sitting right in the middle of her room was a huge overstuffed suitcase that was so full it would hardly close. I had told her to just bring old clothes to wear at the beach. She brought everything.

The two of us sat on the suitcase until it shut. It took both of us to carry it out to the car. My mom must have grinned when she saw us coming. There was Ginny with literally no sense of color coordination, wearing clothes that were ripped, dirty, and too small. And here we were carrying a whole load of those clothes to the beach.

On the way to the cabin Ginny told us how her mom bought everything at secondhand stores. Now I understood all the mismatched, strange-colored, and wrong-sized clothing. Her mother bought whatever size was available that she could afford.

When we got to the cabin, we had to unload everything. Nobody was looking forward to carrying Ginny's bulging suitcase. We finally did get it down the grass hill, down the stairs and into the cabin. Once inside, Ginny opened her suitcase. She had opened only one side when the other side just exploded. Clothes of every description went flying! My sister and I wanted to laugh, but instead we just went around the room picking up Ginny's secondhand clothes.

That night, we didn't lift up the heavy outdoor shades on the front windows of the cabin. The next morning when my mom opened them so we could see the beach, the tide had already gone out. There were only little pools of water left behind in the ripples of the sand. The sun was shining on the water and sand, making it look like a mirror.

Ginny woke up and started yelling, "It snowed! It snowed!" I didn't understand. It was springtime, how could it have snowed? It hadn't. Ginny had never been to the beach before and didn't know that the water came in and out. She thought the water would be there when we woke up. Instead she saw the sun shining on the tide flats and thought it snowed during the night.

I realized then how privileged I was to have had the chance to be at the beach at such an early age. I also realized how lucky I was to have a mom who cared about us. She made sure that we had clean clothes that matched and were the right size. She combed my hair before I could do it myself. Ginny had so little, but she didn't seem to know it. She wasn't unhappy that her mom didn't take care of her or that her clothes were funny - she didn't know that things should be any different. I did.

ASSESSMENTS

Though I had assembled a band of friends by the end of first grade, I hadn't learned how to read or do any of the other first grade level skills well enough. My mom was told to put me in another school. I know now that it was devastating for my mom to hear what they were saying. It wasn't, "Hold her back for a year." It was, "Take her out of here; we can't help her."

I was given labels, but no solutions. I had audio, visual, and motor problems. Maybe they called it dyslexia then; maybe there were even more labels. They could give us the labels, but no one told us what to do about the problems. They could tell my mom to take me out of public schools, but no one could tell her where to put me. They couldn't say how, when, or if I would improve, or if there was a way to get help for me.

I was not aware of exactly what was happening at the time. I knew I wasn't doing very well and that even going to a resource room hadn't stopped my learning problems, although it had helped. But, my mom kept all the assessments from me so that I wouldn't be discouraged.

I already disliked school. Telling me that they said to find another school for me would have made me want to never go back. But my mom kept this information to herself. She fought the battle for me by talking a teacher into keeping me in her class for the next two years. That teacher agreed.

If I hadn't had my mom to speak on my behalf, I don't know where I would be right now. If I had been moved out of a regular school and cast aside, it would have been devastating. Even though I knew that I was having trouble in the regular classroom, staying there was better than being removed and labeled somewhere else.

At the end of my first grade year, my resource room teacher announced that she was leaving. She was going to be moving out of the area. I was very sad; Mrs. Schlosser made school bearable for me and now she was going to leave.

At the end of the year, we had a little party in the resource room. I have a photograph that was taken that day with me standing next to Mrs. Schlosser. In the picture my eyes are facing down, I have a faint smile, and my hands are clasped tightly in front of me. My regular classroom teacher was standing on the other side of Mrs. Schlosser and she, like me, looked strained. It was obvious I was uncomfortable and I'm sure she was, too.

BLUE RIBBONS-RODEOS-LITTLE RED BARNS

The summer after first grade was spent up at our beach cabin. When summer came, we moved up there for about three months. We came back home off and on, but most of time was spent looking under rocks for baby crabs and swimming in the channels on the tide flats.

There was always something to do. We could pick blackberries across the street from our cabin and cherries from the neighbor's tree. My sister and I would pick the berries and my mom would make the pies. We had fresh pie once a week.

My mom found that the best way to protect my sister and me from the local bullies who lived nearby was to let the bullies pick the berries and she would bake pies. We were the only kids on the block who got to know the bullies on a first name basis. You see, they would come over early in the morning carrying buckets of berries. They would sit on our front steps until my mom had finished making the pie. My mom would open the door, hand them forks, pies, and plates. In minutes, the pie was gone.

All the people down the beach were wondering how she was taming the bullies. Little did they know, all it took was a little sugar and flour. From that time on, she was known as the pie lady, and we were the only kids who didn't get our candy stolen while coming back from the store.

That summer my mom first discovered the fair. Someone told her that there was a fair going on during August and that you could enter anything and get a ribbon for it. My mom came back from the town with the good news and we started gathering up things to enter. We gathered up old art projects and made new ones. We made sand candles by pouring colored wax into the sand and letting it harden. A messy project to transport, but definitely worth a first prize blue ribbon. Then there was the great rock art, where you take rocks and sea shells and glue them on to a piece of drift wood. The final touch was to paint eyes on the rocks and shells to bring them to life, and you had at least a second prize red ribbon!

Our projects were judged against those who had been members of 4-H groups for years. They had skills for sewing, baking, growing vegetables, and raising animals - skills that my sister and I couldn't possibly have.

When it came to sewing, my sister did better than I. I couldn't reach the pedal of the machine. My legs dangled while I sat at the picnic table. My mom had to press the pedal to make the machine start and I would run the fabric through. I made a pair of pants from a very simple pattern that year. The fabric had little pink mice on it, and for as long as they lasted, they were my favorite pants. I didn't win any major awards for my pants, but I learned how to sew.

The last thing that I was determined to do was to make bread to enter in the fair. I had watched my mom make homemade bread many times, and I decided that was going to be my ultimate project.

My mom tried, but there was no talking me out of it. She had every reason why I shouldn't do it. I had every reason why I should. Finally she let me make a loaf of bread to enter in the fair.

In the end, my idea proved to be a good one. She helped me measure and stir, and then when it was time to knead the bread, my mom found out that kneading bread was a great pastime for a hyperactive kid. She just put me at the end of our plastic covered picnic table, and I would direct my excess energy towards that dough. I didn't just knead the dough, I beat the tar out of it. My mom thought I had kneaded it so hard that it would surely never rise. But rise it did.

We took every project in on a Thursday morning so the judges could make their decisions; and when the gates opened on Friday, we were first in line. We immediately ran to see all of our art projects; some had blue ribbons, some had red, and some had white. First, second, and third prizes. My sister and I went around counting the blues because they were first prize. There were a few of those and more of the others. We had a good time no matter what ribbons we had.

The next place we visited was the Grange. That's where the baking, canning, sewing, and vegetables were exhibited. I ran in and looked all over for my loaf of bread. I looked and looked for that little loaf, but it was nowhere to be found. After I had searched the whole Grange, I came up to my mom and I was on the verge of tears. "Mom, someone must have eaten my bread."

My mom helped me find the person in charge of the Grange. I went and tugged on the woman's coat. Her name was Marietta, and she didn't even crack a smile when I told her my heartbreaking story of the lost bread. She listened closely and then led me over to a tall glass case. It wasn't like all the other cases or shelves that held exhibits, it was a glass case.

Marietta pointed to the top of the case and there it was. My bread. To my surprise, it didn't have a red ribbon, a blue ribbon, or a white attached to it. My bread, the bread that never should have risen, had a red, white, and blue ribbon attached to it and right in the middle of it, were the words BEST OF FAIR in big gold letters.

I still have that ribbon. It is a little wrinkled and faded, but it is kept with all of the things from my past that are special to me. About a year ago, I was reunited with Marietta when I gave the keynote speech at a 4-H Leaders Forum. Marietta was there and I was able to thank her in front of all her peers and fellow leaders for her kindness. We weren't members of 4-H, we were just a couple of kids from the beach who wanted to enter something in the local fair. Marietta helped us and became our friend over the years. I was grateful to have the chance to thank her and to let her see what had become of the littlest breadmaker.

Usually my sister won everything while I stood in the shadows, but the fair was different. First I won the BEST OF FAIR ribbon for my bread. Then one year I won a ribbon at the style show. To other people, the ribbons were just ribbons. To me, they were the A's I didn't get in school. I still have a book with all those ribbons, and I saved the articles from the local paper that show me holding my first and only style show ribbon.

If you wanted to find me during the three days of the fair, there were only two places you would have to look: the horse show ring or a place called The Little Red Barn. I had been a horse lover from the first time I knew what a horse was. Everyone said, "She'll outgrow it," but I never did. I sat for hours in the heat and smell of the horse show ring with every fly in the universe congregating around my head. I never moved, I didn't even shift. I was mesmerized by the beauty and the strength of these animals. I watched the riders and memorized each move and command that they gave their horses. When I finally got a chance to ride for the first time, I rode like I had been doing it all my life.

I would watch and listen. Sometimes, I would even sneak into the back lot where all of the horses and riders would go when they were in between shows. I would slip through a fence and hope that I would meet someone and get to pet their horse. I would walk among the trailers and watch everyone grooming and saddling their horses. Just being among those riders was heaven for me. Being there somehow removed any bad thoughts or worries. Each year, I would go back. Each year, I had more going on in my life, and seeing the horses took me away and back to a time when things were easier.

I remember one year I was about nine years old, watching a little girl and her pony win the highest prize for her division. She had long hair and a cowgirl outfit that was all perfectly matched. I had her picked right from the beginning. She had perfect posture and commanded her pony with ease. Watching her made me dream I was riding off into the sunset on my pony. I had that dream a lot; the older I became the more detailed it became - having a pony in my backyard and a closet full of every color of overalls that could be made. That was my way of escaping, to be on a horse where I had control and power.

If I wasn't at the horse show ring, there was only one other place to look. I found The Little Red Barn on my own and it was exactly like it sounds. Inside, bales of hay were used as chairs. Kids of all ages would be dropped off by their parents, and we would sit and listen to a storyteller read stories from the Bible. It was usually women who told these stories while sitting on a hay bale with us. After the story was told, we would all bow our heads and pray. During the prayer, the storyteller or teacher would ask if anyone of us would like to give our hearts to the Lord. I was saved at least five times a day, each day that the fair was going on.

It was assumed that when the story was told and the prayer was over, that the group that was in the barn would leave to allow the next group to come in. I wonder what they thought when they opened the barn door and I just sat there. I was a permanent fixture on my bale of hay and knew all the storytellers by name. Whenever there was a break in the horse show action, I was in that barn door with lightning speed.

I always found comfort in Bible stories. I found comfort in knowing that God was so much bigger than me. I knew the story of the day at the Little Red Barn and could listen to it over and over again and never be bored. There was a Father in Heaven so great that he could forgive me for my imperfections. I am grateful for learning about God early, and am grateful that there was such a thing as The Little Red Barn. It was better than Sunday school because I could hear the stories rather than read them, and it was better than church because I was not sitting in a pew behind a Sunday hat. On that bale of hay among people who only knew my first name, I could see and hear and I learned.

SECOND AND THIRD GRADE

I entered Miss Driscoll's class with some reservations. However, the first day I learned I had nothing to fear. Her class was much different than any other I had been in. It was quieter. I don't know how she did it with thirty kids, but she managed. Her manner was soft; she didn't yell or move quickly. She acted and reacted in the same ways that my resource room teacher did. She didn't do things fast and loud; if she had, she wouldn't have been able to reach me. Instead she reminded me of things, her directions were clear and in order, and she would repeat herself if necessary.

She knew what others had said about me. She may have even been in on the meeting when my mom was told to remove me from school. No matter what she knew, she didn't give up on me. She took me into her class and expected me to do well. I knew that she cared because she looked at me when she talked to me. She would compliment me when I did well. I was so hungry for praise and, in her calm voice, she would give me acceptance and rewards. These rewards lowered the pressure that I had previously felt at school and allowed me the freedom to do my best at my own pace.

The first year that I was in her class I didn't make any astonishing strides. She learned early that my energy had to be channeled or I would be in trouble most of the time. She would constantly remind me of what I was supposed to be doing and, in time, I learned to remind myself. She also helped keep me out of trouble by keeping me busy. She was one of the first teachers who allowed me to help her in the classroom. While everyone else was worried that I would get in the way or get into trouble, she believed in me and on special occasions I got to help her.

In her class the schedule was constant. She was consistent and also organized. Each of these factors was necessary for me to learn. Because I knew what was coming up and what was going to happen,

I asked fewer questions and was less jittery and nervous. Because everything was organized and predictable, I felt more in control and less overwhelmed than in my other classrooms. It was also quiet in her room so I was able to focus my attention better and consequently learned much more.

I grew to love and respect Miss Driscoll so much so that if she ever got mad at me, I thought the world would fall in. I loved her and her gentle ways. I wanted to please her because she believed in me. In her class I was not the hyperactive kid with learning disabilities. I was just a kid. I began to act the part. As another great teacher, Jaime Escalante, said in the movie Stand and Deliver, "Kids will rise to the level of expectations." I did.

Looking back on the two years spent in Miss Driscoll's class I now see that I learned many things, but there were three things in particular which would help me to not only learn, but prepare to learn, for the rest of my years in school.

First, Miss Driscoll constantly reminded me and put me back on focus when I got distracted and went off track. She didn't yell. Yelling upset and distressed me. She talked to me in a calm voice, telling me in repetition what was to be done, and what was going to happen. It was these reminders in repetition that worked for me.

In time, I learned to focus and concentrate on what she was saying, repeat it in repetition to myself and in turn I asked fewer questions, was less distracted and didn't distract those around me.

Second, she looked at me when she talked to me. She knew that I had to see her face, lips and hand movements to make the connection with what she was saying. Other people had said I just wasn't listening. The truth is, they just weren't looking at me when they talked and I couldn't understand them.

She also moved me to the front of the room rather than moving me to the back. She knew that having people in front of me was just another obstacle for me to get through to get to the words she was saying. She put me up in front and I was less distracted, and I could see and hear everything clearly.

Third, the key to helping learning disabled children survive and be successful is to teach them how to be organized. As I said before, her room was organized and constant. Because of this, I calmed down and could go to work and focus my energy on what I was learning. I became part of the organized pattern of her classroom just as I had become part of the disorganized pattern in my former classrooms.

Not long ago I saw Miss Driscoll. She hadn't aged at all. I said, "I guess I was a real handful, wasn't I?" She said, "Oh, Shari, you weren't a bad girl, but a student who tried really hard." She treated me just as a kid who had to try hard. With her, and for her, I did try hard and I did succeed.

THE FIFTY STATES

Even though Miss Driscoll seemingly did everything she could to help me succeed, every now and then there was a miscommunication. I'm sure that there was more than one incident that left her shaking her head, but as for me, I will never forget trying to learn the states and the capitals.

At some point during the year, we had an assignment to learn the fifty states and capitals. Projects like this one always seemed like a mountain to me. I could memorize my Disney records, but I had not had the same luck with memorizing things that were not put to music. I was wondering if I would be able to read a map and be able to remember it all.

That night I went to the corner drugstore to get a workbook on the fifty states, but they didn't have one. I realize now that a workbook probably wouldn't have helped me anyway. Reading wasn't my best form of learning. Instead, we found a puzzle that had large pieces. Each piece of the puzzle was a state and had the capital located on it. When you put it all together, you had a map of the United States.

I took that puzzle home and my sister helped me put it together. I spent the next two weeks in the back room of our house, on the floor, with my puzzle. I started lifting up each piece one by one. I would visualize what the first row of states were. There was Washington, Oregon, and California. I would lift up the Washington piece, close my eyes and visualize where it went and what the capital was. I memorized its shape and which state was near it so that I would have a connection when I went to fill out the test.

Do you see the difference here? Other kids could memorize the states and capitals by reading a map or a list of them, but for me, it was not enough just to read. I had to put a visual image, a touch, and a sound with the words. I had to touch the puzzle pieces, taking them in and out of the puzzle one by one to reinforce the image. I had to say the words out loud and visualize the map in my head. I had to use all of my senses to grasp the information.

I put the map in a mental image in my head. I would go down the first row of states on the west coast. Then I would move over to the next line of states, moving from left to right. Some states were lined up horizontally, some were in a vertical line and some weren't lined up at all. It took me longer to learn those that weren't in some kind of line or pattern.

Even how the names sounded in relation to each other helped me to learn the information. I didn't just say the states and the capitals, I would sort of "rap" them. I would lean over my map, close my eyes and start naming the states and capitols to a sort of rap beat. Just as with the A, B, C's, without singing them I wouldn't remember them. Without putting a beat or rhythm to the words, the states and capitals didn't stay in my memory.

It took a lot of time and a lot of repetition before I thought I could look at the test and visualize where every thing on the map should be. I would just get it memorized, then I would come back to it the next day and I would have to re-learn some of the states from the day before. Little by little, I would add one more state to the map in my head. By the time the test arrived, I had my visual picture in perfect order.

On test day, I looked at the blank test in front of me and started to panic. I wondered if I would be able to remember what I had worked so hard on. I closed my eyes and pretended that I was back at home, sitting on my knees, picking up puzzle pieces and then putting them back as I said the name out loud. I went back to that time when there was no pressure.

The panic started to wear off, and pretty soon my mental picture was coming back to me. I started filling out the test, state by state, line by line. Even though I knew a certain state over on the other side of the map, I didn't fill it in. I filled each row of states out just as I had practiced on my own. I have found that if you have a pattern to how you do something, it is much better to stick with it. If I had started filling out the states randomly, my mental picture and pattern would have been disrupted.

Just like with cleaning, I found that my learning patterns had to be rigid and repetitious. I would try to deviate from my rigid patterns and rituals and learn like other kids, but it was then that I would fail. There were days that I would become frustrated with the long processes and tight controls that I had to follow to learn, and I would want to be free like the other kids in my classroom. In time, I learned to put up with the patterns and rigidity of it all. As long as I learned, that was all that mattered.

When I was finished with the test, I thought I had done so well. Everything was filled out, I had remembered all the states and the capitols and had them each in the right place.

When we got our tests back, mine was covered with red ink. I only got a score of about 50 percent. I thought there must have been some mistake. It was then that I realized that I had learned all of the states and capitals -I just hadn't learned how to spell them.

You might be thinking that it is impossible for someone to learn all the states and the capitals but not learn how to spell them. Not if you are an eight year old learning disabled child. You couldn't assume anything with me. The teacher assumed that I would learn how to spell the states and capitols when I learned their location on the map. I never did.

There must be times when parents and teachers and even brothers and sisters believe that you're not listening. How could you not learn how to spell them? Why don't you follow directions? Why are you asking me the same question for the hundredth time? Spelling things out and repeating yourself is the only way to work with children like me. When I was a child you had to look me in the eye to see if I was really hearing you, or if I was just nodding my head hoping to please you with my understanding. In time, I knew what I had to do to learn, but when I was little, I needed the direction and guidance of a teacher. I needed a hand on my shoulder or the teacher's voice to remind me what we were doing, to tell me the directions again and to put me back on track.

No, it isn't unusual for a learning disabled child to miss some of the most obvious things, to seemingly go through life with only one eye open. I wasn't testing anybody, I was just dyslexic. I wasn't naive, I just needed things to be laid out in an organized and sometimes repetitive way. Even then, I sometimes made mistakes.

LEARNING HOW TO READ

As my third year of elementary school progressed, I became better and better at reading, but my progress was gradual. Other kids were reading circles around me, but in the quiet caring atmosphere of my third grade classroom, I improved.

For one thing, nobody was standing over me with a stern face waiting for me to progress quickly. I was not embarrassed or pressured, but there were expectations of me. My teacher was involved with me. I felt special because of her attention but I never felt that she was singling me out as different from the rest. In that atmosphere, reading became a possibility for me.

There were still problems, of course. The words still looked like jumbled bunches of letters. Each word was an obstacle and I had to sound it out letter by letter, and each sentence word by word. I would sound out each letter and put the word together, but there wasn't immediate recognition with words. "And," "or," and "the," I knew immediately. But most of the other words I had to sound out.

My reading was slow and deliberate, my voice was monotone. I had to concentrate so hard on the words that I couldn't add emotion to my voice. I did not follow the lines on a page with my eyes, I followed with my head. When I was reading silently, I moved my lips, reading each word quietly to myself. I preferred to read in dim light. The brighter the light, the more trouble I had with concentration. Bright light also seemed to affect my dyslexic symptoms relating to reading. In bright light the words jumped around more than usual, and my eyes couldn't get focused. I felt I wanted to put my hand on the page to stop the words from moving.

Even when I mastered reading, I realized that I could read but I didn't absorb any of it. I could read a book several times and start to understand it, but an hour later could not remember what I had read. I could remember seemingly pointless facts about characters but not remember their names or where the story took place. If someone was talking next to me while I was reading, I would incorporate the facts of the story with whatever they were saying in their conversation.

One of the most interesting things I learned about myself was that it was more comfortable for me to read from right to left than from left to right. I mean it actually felt more normal than the way that I had always been taught (left to right). When I was reading, it often felt like I was going against the grain by reading from left to right. Another interesting thing is that when I was reading, I tended to lead with my weak eye, rather than read with a balance of both eyes. My right eye is actually worse than my left, but for some reason I preferred to lead with it anyway.

This emphasis caused my right eye to become tired much easier and reading often made me sleepy. Once again, light was always a factor. If the lights were dim, I didn't have to work as hard to keep the letters still on the page and my eyes didn't become as tired.

In the beginning of the year, a new reading program was introduced. Boxes of specially selected books were brought into our class, and put into sectioned cases in the back of our room. The books were numbered one to sixty. We could go back and select a book, read it and then take a test on it. If we passed the test we could move on to the next book. We didn't have to read the books in order, but we had to read all the books to finish the program. As we went higher in number, the books were longer and more difficult.

Like everyone else, I chose a book. I read it, took the test and went on to the next book. I thought that I would hate it. I was surprised. I found myself looking forward to reading time so that I could get through another book. I had hated reading before, but there was something different this time. It was becoming easier to read. What everyone else had learned in first grade, I was just starting to accomplish. The dyslexia wasn't gone, but my concentration was better in this quiet room. The stories were interesting and the books were short, which helped to make me feel that I was making progress.

Earlier, I had been so caught up in sounding out the words that I didn't understand the story nor could I remember it. By the middle of the year, I was actually reading, slowly but consistently. It wasn't as halting as it had been before, the words were starting to become words rather than black dots on a page. More than that, I started to like to read. Prior to this time, reading was such a long process that I was frustrated, therefore I hated it. Now that I saw a little progress and had a pattern to follow (read a book, take a test, read the next book, etc.), I was encouraged. It was a program that I could do on my own, and it became a personal challenge to get through the books.

I was one of the few people in our class to finish the whole reading program. I felt so good about that. It was a personal victory for me as a third grader. I was reading for the first time in my life. I had finished the program that other kids, kids who were smarter than I, hadn't. I knew that my teacher would be happy, but I experienced a pride in myself that I had never felt before. I can remember putting that last book on the shelf and thinking, "I did it." It was one of the few times between preschool and seventh grade that I felt good about something at school.

By the end of my third year, my reading scores had changed dramatically. I still had trouble with spelling and comprehension, but I was reading. I believe it was this improvement in reading that made it possible for me to stay in public schools in the years to follow. My third grade teacher couldn't keep me in her class forever; eventually I would have to move on. But thanks to her, I learned how to read.

CHAPTER 6

After third grade, I continued to stay in public schools, but I was no longer given any help through a resource room or other special services. I was glad that I wasn't separated from the rest of the class, yet I was struggling so much in school that I hoped someone would help me.

In third grade, my teacher had somehow known how to keep me on track. By fourth grade, my teacher was good, but was unaware of the time and attention that I needed so desperately. There was noise in the classroom all the time, and the pattern and repetition that I had grown accustomed to was now replaced by a faster pace. In this different environment, any positive study skills that I did pick up in Miss Driscoll's class were left behind. Now, instead of keeping up or even moving forward, it was just a matter of survival.

I was behind and struggling; but because I could read, it was as if they sent down a decree that said, "If she can read, then she doesn't need our help anymore." As with so many kids, I was slipping through the cracks. As long as   teachers were willing to take me into their classrooms, as long as I wasn't a major behavior problem, and as long as I wasn't too far behind, I was passed along.

We were facing many obstacles similar to what parents and kids are facing today. Even though the law now says that learning disabled children are to be given an appropriate education in the public school system, unfortunately due to lack of funding, sometimes the programs don't meet the requirements of this mandate. A school may have a program, but it may take a long time before the required diagnostic tests can be given. If a child does make it into the program, he still has to deal with the separation and stigma associated with it. And because these programs are so overburdened, a child who could use help today often doesn't get it because he is on the borderline of qualifying. There are problems with all of these scenarios but the worst is being unable to qualify. A child may not be far enough behind today, but in a year he will be. By then he will have been through another year of failure and embarrassment. A year later when the system does deem him qualified, the child has been beaten down and has lost his spirit to learn.

The students are damaged by this mixed-up system, and parents become angry and frustrated as a result. It's their child who is coming home from school crying. The parents don't know how to help. They are sure that the school has all the answers. But teachers are victims of this system, too. All teachers find it frustrating to see the needs of any student go unmet. But with a lack of resources, it is sometimes virtually impossible to meet the needs of any student and especially special needs students.

Teachers know that if these special needs students don't get help, these kids may never reach their potential. No teacher likes to see this happen to kids, but this problem is even more intensified for resource room teachers. They know why so many parents seem pushy, aggressive and driven on behalf of their children. They know what kind of system we have, and what happens to kids if they don't get help. They also watch the many faces that walk in and out of their doors every day and hope, as the children's parents do, that they can reach them.

I hear teachers and administrators complain about parents who come to school and complain about a program, lack of resources, or mistreatment of their child. To me, it isn't any big mystery. If you love your child, you will fight for him. As a parent you may be overprotective, but you also have watched your child struggle and scrape to function in school. If the system can't help, a parent faces the question of who will with pain, frustration, and worry. Educators must be sensitive to this.

In my opinion, early intervention is the key. Get children the help they need as early as possible. The longer you have to develop the skills that you need to survive when you have a learning problem, the less likely you are to give up. That means teachers must learn to recognize learning problems in the mainstream classroom and act quickly to get help for that child.

There are districts which have put learning disabled children in the mainstream classroom and use resource room teachers in the classrooms to help those students who have specific problems. The program lowers the stigma on the child, which in turn makes him more likely to succeed. It lowers the burden on the mainstream teacher who has a fellow teacher there to help with the extra needs of the learning disabled child, and it also decreases the burden of responsibility that the resource room teacher has. This system of mainstreaming and providing help within the classroom is one which, if implemented correctly, could work for everyone.

That is now. But when I sat in my fourth grade classroom, there was nowhere for me to go and few who knew how to help me.

MULTIPLYING MY PROBLEMS

Each year brought new things to learn. And each year we seemed to stray farther and farther away from the concrete learning which worked best for me, moving towards abstract learning in which you had to see things in your head. There were new symbols and new meanings to words. By the end of each year I would just start to catch on to what they were teaching, but the next year would bring something new.

When I speak about concrete learning, I mean the kind of learning

90

that you can see and touch. I could see the three apples and the three oranges being put together for addition, and I could see the two apples being taken away for subtraction. Now they were saying an "x" means times. I couldn't understand that symbol. I couldn't understand why 2x2=4. How did you get it, why can't we just go 2+2? That I could see, that I could understand.

By fourth grade we were required to learn the multiplication tables. It was my longest and toughest learning experience yet. I tried memorizing them and I tried writing them out, but still the numbers wouldn't stick. It seemed that because I couldn't understand the meaning of the multiplication symbol "x," my mind couldn't accept that 5x8=40.

Some people can just accept a new symbol or a new fact and assume that it is true. I couldn't assume; I had to ask why it is this way. My teacher would try to explain again and again why 5x8=40. "Well, Shari, because five eights adds up to forty." He would just finish explaining this to me and I would be up at the desk again asking him, "Why?"

Asking me to memorize the times tables was hard enough. Then they expected me to be able to take a timed test where the teacher stood at the front of the room with a stopwatch, and we were supposed to complete a paper filled with multiplication tables in the allotted time. When the teacher said, "Go," my brain would stop. I would try to figure out the problems one by one in long form. Since 5x8 means five eights added up, I would add them. You can see why when the teacher said, "Stop," I had only three or four of the twenty problems finished.

I wish I knew why pressure made the test, or anything for that matter, that much harder. The only thing that I can say is that pressure made me make more mistakes and made me unable to recall even the most familiar information. With practice, I have learned to deal with this problem. Experience teaches you how to gain control. In fourth grade I didn't know how to keep the information from disappearing during a test or how to block the noise and hold my concentration when the stopwatch was on. It's one thing when the numbers were all there on the page or the apples and oranges told you how many were there and how many were being taken away, but the times tables required memorization, recall at a moment's notice, and understanding for things that were represented by a symbol rather than shown or pictured on a page.

There were times when I sensed my teacher's frustration when I repeatedly asked him the same questions. I was not his only student; there was classroom full of us. He tried not to lose control. He was too busy, so inevitably he would rush through the information with me again and I would go back to my seat as bewildered as before. He was not the problem - I liked him - it was the times tables that were the problem. People didn't know how to teach the times tables to a kid like me, so we both ended up being frustrated.

I would dread daily math time. The other students got frustrated with me because I was prone to ask questions of those around me. They wondered why they should tell me what the answer to 5x8 was when they had just told me the answer to that question five minutes ago. Besides, we were supposed to have learned the tables three months prior. Yes, I was behind as always. I felt dumb and I was as tired of asking questions as other people were of answering them.

This is the mainstream teacher's dilemma today: Who do I help, the mainstream kids or the learning disabled kids? I have had people ask me time and time again, "Why should we have learning disabled kids in our classroom if they can't do what all the other kids can do? They just take up time that could be going to all the other students."

People have asked this question for years and some have even tried to prove that learning disabled kids cannot be helped in the public school setting, if at all. They prove it by expecting a learning disabled student to have problems. They prove it by being inflexible regarding the form in which a child is allowed to learn. Without any alternatives, the child doesn't learn, so their theory is proven.

The opposite can also be proven. The key is to help the child develop the skills to figure out the problem on his own. The child then becomes independent and is able to remain in the mainstream classroom system. By using patterning, repetition, teaching the child how to self-talk his way through a problem, teaching other children to help those around them, any student can survive and even thrive in the mainstream.

A learning disabled student will ask more questions, take more of the teacher's time and misunderstand directions most of the time. However, a teacher can make it possible for him to learn simply by looking him straight in the eye and saying it is possible. Offering encouragement and reassurance frees up his mind to learn. Then when you break it down or show them a different way of working out a problem that will be more concrete or will illustrate the problem in a different light, you will see that child succeed.

Only a small portion of the resources that I have just listed were made available to me in my fourth grade classroom. Instead, I found my source of help in a very unlikely place.

There were kids in my class who wondered what was wrong with me, but there were also one or two who protected me as I had protected my little misfit friends in first grade. There was one girl who sat next to me, who was half my size with dark eyes and a soft voice barely above a whisper. She would watch me during math and wonder why I couldn't do the problems. There were times when I would be on the verge of tears because I didn't understand, and she would pat me on the shoulder and explain it to me.

It was through my struggles in math that we became friends. Each day she helped me in some form or another. For her, she was just answering a simple question. For me, it meant having a tutor sitting next to me, walking me through the hardest subject. I had to lean close to hear her when she spoke, but her words were clear. She spoke slowly and deliberately, as if she knew I needed more time. She would explain each step of the math problem and go over it again if need be.

It became a given that at recess we would go out on the playground and walk together. We weren't talking about dolls or our weekend plans, we were going over the times tables. I don't know how it started. I guess she knew I needed help and neither one of us had many other friends, so it gave us something to do.

There we were. She would start with 2x1, and go through the two's. She would give me a problem and I would say it out loud. Each week I would add another number and practice the times tables for that number at recess. The bigger the number, the harder it was to learn but my friend was never impatient. I worked on memorization on my own, but her help was irreplaceable.

My goal was to get all the way through the times tables from one through ten. By the time I reached seven I thought I would never make it. Some numbers were my enemies. Five, seven, eight and nine were the numbers that I hated the most. I don't know why, but I always seemed to get more confused with those numbers. 6x7 and 7x6 were like two different questions to me. If you asked me those two equations, I would probably come up with two different answers. To me, they sounded different so they were different. Certain number combinations like 8x9, 5x6, and 7x6 were hardest for me to remember. Those were the ones that my friend would quiz me on.

One day it all came together. It wasn't that all of a sudden the "x" symbol made sense or those particular numbers were no longer my enemies. The bottom line was that with repetitive learning, I had finally managed to memorize the times tables facts. Understanding them was not my concern. Again, it was survival. Get what you can get. Hold on to what will get you through and leave the rest to the other kids who aren't learning disabled.

We were on the playground, when all the repetition finally paid off. My friend looked at me, I looked at her, and we both yelled with excitement. She had been in on this from the very beginning and she was almost as happy as I was. It was as if the information

93

finally crossed the imaginary boundary in my brain to the place where I could understand and retrieve the information. That's the best way to explain it. There was this imaginary line that always seemed to be changing to a different place. Some information would be easily accepted and could cross the border in my mind almost immediately. Other types of information would not cross the border even after many attempts to learn it.

I couldn't contain my excitement - I had to tell someone. My teacher was on playground duty that day, so I dragged my poor friend behind me until we found him. For all the times that he wondered why he couldn't get the multiplication tables into my head, for the times that he masked his impatience with me, I had to show him that I finally had it figured out. Without time for him to realize what happened, I said, "Listen to this." I then proceeded to recite all the times tables from two through ten.

I think back on how funny it must have been for me to come up and start saying the times tables to my teacher out of the blue. I couldn't have waited; it was that important to me. My teacher was surprised, glad, and probably a little confused. I'm sure he wondered how I finally learned all of them. When I stopped asking questions of him, he had moved on to help other kids, my problems were not as visible to him. He had placed me in the back of his mind, now here I was rattling off my toughest assignment.

I didn't necessarily learn the times tables from him, nor did I receive special services or intervention for my problems while in his class. I did get caring and patience whenever possible, I got his sense of humor in the face of adversity (he had a way of laughing that made school work a little easier to bear), and I was never embarrassed or singled out in his class. I am grateful to him, if not for what he did, more so for what he didn't do. And I will never forget my little friend, who out of the goodness of her heart took the time to get those times tables over the bridge into a place where I could understand them.

Learning those multiplication tables was very important to me. It is a basic skill I needed, just like reading. In most areas I was academically at least a year behind kids my age, so I learned the second lesson of survival: prioritize. Spelling was secondary to being able to learn what a word meant and being able to use it correctly in speech. The math story problems were secondary to the addition and the multiplication. And reading seemed to be more important than everything. I was behind in all my subjects, so I had to pick the things that I needed the most and focus all of my energy into them.

I realize now that had my teacher said, "If you can't learn the times tables now, you can't be in my class," I might have thought it impossible. Whether he made a conscious decision to allow me

94

to go along at my own pace, or because he didn't have another alternative, I did not give up and eventually I learned.

VIOLIN LESSONS

Even though my sister and I were different, I hoped that someday I would be like her. I wore her hand-me-down clothes with pride and I tried to act and talk like her. I even tried to write like her, copying her slant and loopy style closely. She was not an easy act to follow, but I kept trying.

My sister started taking violin lessons through a school program during her fourth grade year. So when I reached fourth grade, of course I wanted to take violin lessons, too. My mom's rule with any kind of lessons was that if you want to take something, you have to give it a year. If after the year is over you want to quit, then you can. Shawn put in her year and I was determined to put in mine.

I took the lessons from a lady who, like so many, wanted to be in control in her class. The chairs were in a row, the kids sat quietly in that row, and the class was to proceed without interruption. I never did very well in tightly kept rooms, there was never enough room for my differences.

I cut my nails when I first entered violin class, but they were never short enough for my teacher. She would often make comments like, "Miss Rusch, didn't we talk about cutting those nails?" I would vow to cut them, but at the next lesson the same comment would be made. If it wasn't my nails, it was something else. If she wasn't mad at me, she didn't say anything to me and being ignored hurt just as much.

I wasn't learning how to play the violin any faster than I learned how to read. Reading music was like reading another language and my brain functioned (or didn't function) as usual. Think of all the things that you must coordinate to play music. Your hands, fingers, and arms must do what your brain tells you to do when you read the little black notes on the little black lines. With my lack of hand-eye coordination and poor small motor skills, it seemed that I was fighting an uphill battle to hold the violin and bow, read the notes and then make my fingers and hands interpret them correctly. Believe me, I hit more wrong notes than right.

I think my teacher thought that there was a simple solution to my problem, and I guess she thought she would remedy the situation by making an example of me. One day, my teacher called me up to the front of the room and she took her nail clippers out of her bag, took one of my hands, and started cutting my nails. One by one, the nails were cut. I didn't want to cry in front of everyone, but the tears were in my eyes. My nails were one

95

of my few features that I thought were pretty.

My teacher didn't even know me, she didn't know that the reason I couldn't play the violin had very little to do with my nails. She just reached in her bag and embarrassed me in front of the class. If she had looked a little farther, she would have realized that I couldn't read music. I guessed or memorized the sound of every piece that we learned. But she never looked that deeply. I made her uncomfortable. I made her mad because I didn't catch on right away.

I was afraid of her and, at the same time, I was angry with her. I stayed in the class until the year was over, but I never liked my teacher and I didn't improve because my teacher never cared about me.

The spring concert held no big surprises. My parents sat in the audience with everyone else listening as we tuned up and prepared for the concert. Our teacher had each violinist play a note to get in tune with each other. She went down the row and each student played the note right on cue. My instructor got to me and, try as I might, I couldn't hit the note. The more she stared at me and the harder I tried, the worse it got. She could have passed over me, but she refused. She stared at me, and my parents sat in agony praying that I would just hit the note and get it over with. I can almost see them, leaning forward in their seats and wishing they could pluck the darn thing for me. They couldn't have wanted it any more than myself, but my fingers just wouldn't cooperate. I think this whole scene would make a great anti-perspirant commercial.

Finally, I played the note and heaved a sigh of relief; my teacher's eyes were off me now and on to another student. My mom never forgot that concert and neither have I. After that year, I turned in my rented violin and was glad to have that particular musical experience over with. In the end, my teacher also got what she wanted. I didn't sign up for violin lessons the next year.

These years in school were frustrating and it was continually confirmed through all those around me, that I was different. By fourth grade I was beginning to feel that just singing a song, making beds, and even the strides that I had made in school would never make up for all of the things that I wasn't. Insecurities are part of growing up, but with each year my insecurities became greater and greater.

I was behind in school and didn't have many friends. I felt weak around authority, I wanted praise from my teachers and at the same time, I feared I would never be able to please them. School was becoming increasingly difficult and I was wondering what would happen to me. I was in the public school system but honestly didn't know if I was going to be able to stay there, let alone go out into the world with the brain that I had. Social situations were always difficult, with overwhelming noise and multiple conversations overloading my brain and making me tired. School left me disinterested, frustrated, and hungry for praise.

DAD

My dad wondered how to deal with me. I don't think he wanted to know the assessments and the labels that were placed on me. I was his child and to know that I wasn't succeeding in school would in some way reflect on him. My problems were not his fault, I was just born that way and yet, I think he felt responsible.

I don't have lots of memories of my father from when I was little; my dad was working a lot and trying to establish himself in business. That kept him away quite a bit. I knew very little about him, his personality or his feelings. I knew him as I would know an idol or a hero, looking up at him, seeing what was on the outside, and loving him because he was my father. What I really wanted was to have talks with him, to get close to him and know him as only a daughter could.

My father was a good man who worked hard and, together with my mom, supported us. I know this now, but when I was little, he was a distant person. It seemed that he liked to keep to himself and could love without a hoopla or parade. But because he was quiet, there were times when I thought he didn't love me at all.

I was a needy child. I needed praise and demonstrative love more than most kids. As much as I needed his love, I know there were times when my dad didn't know what to do and was unsure how to deal with me. Before we knew much about learning disabilities there was no promise that I was going to do better in school or how far I would even go. He heard the same assessments as my mom and he, too, must have wondered about my future. I always got the feeling that he believed it was easier not to deal with this unusual child than to have to deal with the emotions and needs that I had.

I was not Shawn. I couldn't follow the line or fit into the mold - not for the first grade teacher, the violin teacher, or my dad. Yet, people expected me to conform. Shawn found a way to get close to my dad. I didn't for a long time.

MEMORIES

One of my favorite memories of my father is of his green and white checked pants that he wore when he mowed the lawn. After mowing, he would sit on the porch with my mom next to him. Watching them together made me feel good because I thought they would always be together.

I remember the mornings when my dad would drive my sister and me to school. There were some dogs in our neighborhood whose ritual was to come over to our house early in the morning, tip over our garbage cans, and spread trash all over the place. My dad wouldn't swear out loud, he would just mutter a multitude of unspeakables under his breath while he picked up the garbage. My sister and I couldn't help laughing as he muttered like "Precious Pup," a Saturday morning cartoons character that was popular at that time.

I remember every time we went outside he would say, "Button up your coat." I was always a little slow, so he would sigh, reach down, zip the zipper on my coat, and pull up my hood.

I remember how I worried about him during the anti-smoking campaign at school. I cried and had nightmares at the thought of losing my father because he smoked. My mom finally had to send him into my room one night to tell me that he wasn't going to die of lung cancer. I wanted to believe him, but I knew if he kept smoking, something terrible could happen. I continued to worry until he finally stopped smoking years later.

I always wanted to please my dad. Once, I decided to make him breakfast. I had the cereal with milk up to the brim and a big glass of orange juice all ready to present to him. Adorned with a smile and my pajamas, I brought in the tray. It was at that point that I tripped and sent all of the contents of the tray flying onto my dad, redecorating my parents' bedroom with cornflakes.

I really hated these moments. It was like when I was told not to laugh in church and all of a sudden everything was hilarious. Or the time that my grandma made a casserole with peas in it and in my booming voice I said, "I hate peas!" My dad gave me a light kick under the table and I realized that I had done it again. Yes, those were the times that really assured me that I was not going to be the apple of my father's eye. My dad didn't have to say anything, I knew from his look or his silence. I wanted to be quickly transformed into the perfect child.

I got in trouble a lot as a child, from just about everyone. But when my dad got mad at me, it was different. I remember each time vividly. The only time my dad ever spanked me was the time that I wrote on the back of my sister's paper turkey that she had made at school. It was a simple mistake. My sister wanted justice, my dad spanked me, and I cried, and I cried, and I cried. It wasn't the spanking that bothered me, it was the fact that my dad spanked me. I only wanted to please him, and he was mad at me. I could take a spanking from my mom. She was always telling me that she loved me, so it all balanced out. When Dad got mad at me, it made everything unbalanced. I couldn't stand not pleasing my father.

My feelings concerning my dad tended to be exaggerated. I needed him so much that every little thing, every little emotion that was at all tied to him, was so important to me. Even a small thing like a spanking from him, or losing a gift that he had given me, could make me feel that at any moment I would lose him forever.

My dad gave me a special stuffed teddy bear once. It was one of the few and only gifts that I saw him pick out just for me. I treasured it as if it were gold. My mother had given me many presents, but it was his that I clung to.

One day, we were taking things to a flea market to sell. My mom suggested that I gather up the stuffed animals that made me sneeze and get rid of them. I brought along the bear that my father had given me to keep me company.

While I was getting lemonade with my sister, the bear was accidentally sold. I cried for days. It was just a bear but it was from my father, and I couldn't stand the thought that is was gone. I loved my father so much, but I didn't think that he loved me. In my mind that bear was my only link to him.

I used to go to bed at night and cry about that lost bear. At first I thought I was crying because my favorite bear was gone. Now I realize I was crying because I never really knew my father.

My mom was devoted to my father and we always learned to respect him as the man of the house. Whatever my dad wanted to do, we did. We were always taught to support him and give him respect. It was a sign of the changing times that my mom was working as hard as my father. The difference was that she was also taking care of us, as well as taking care of the house. She assumed all the roles, and my sister and I never questioned it. My mom made us feel very loved and when my dad was home, it was a bonus.

I rarely heard them argue, but I knew when there was tension between them. As with everything else, my mother would cover the problems with sugar so that my sister and I wouldn't worry. I knew things weren't perfect; I knew that there were differences between them; and I knew that sometimes there were tensions between Mom and Dad but nothing seemed really bad as long as they were together.

In my muddled quest to get through school, I missed or should I say refused to see the fights and tensions that meant divorce. I saw things through rose-colored glasses because it was more comfortable than seeing the truth. Just as making the bed first thing in the morning and following my daily routine of rituals helped me to organize my mind and spirit, knowing that my family was together gave me my purpose when there wasn't one. My need for family made me put together my forever box and cling to its contents. My mom covered up anything that would expose my parents' problems. The rest I just refused to see.

I could not face the possibility of disruption. The very thought that my parents might get a divorce sent me into panic. My life at school was all the disruption and disorganization that I could take. I wanted to keep things in order, change made me afraid. I also feared the loss of my father because I didn't know him and I needed him. Divorce might mean that I would never know him or share the relationship with him that I longed for.

I wouldn't face divorce in my family and yet, it was happening around me at school. The boom of divorce and latch key children had not hit its high point yet, but many of the kids that I had started school with were now children of divorce. I remember one girl in particular. She was a little more worldly-wise than I would ever be in the fourth grade. There was just something about her that made me feel that she was a little on the wild side - after all, she had pierced ears.

Her parents had been divorced early in her life and she had been living in a single parent household with her mother working and dating different men. That seemed like the wild side to me. She had many stories that I would listen to like they were a drama rather than real life - stories of her mom's boyfriends, and how she would come home and take care of herself until her mom got home from work. I couldn't relate to it. I looked at her and felt superior somehow because I didn't want to believe that divorce would ever happen to my family.

On the playground, she would tell me about her family. I don't know what made me say it, but all of a sudden I said to her, "My family is never going to get a divorce. My parents love each other and get along just great. That will never happen to us."

I wasn't thinking that in some way my declaration might hurt my friend's feelings. Instead, I think I was saying it just to reassure myself that it couldn't happen. To say it out loud was like affirming it to myself that I would never be alone.

My sister understood what was taking place at home. She could read through the adoring smile of my mother's face and the flat silence of my father to know that there was something very wrong. She heard the fights at night that I either slept through or pretended not to hear. It must have hurt her to know that something was wrong, yet at the same time, it gave her a chance to prepare for what was inevitable.

One day my dad was just gone. I had no warning and was completely unprepared when my mom told us. But where and for how long? I had so many questions. Were they going to divorce or might they get back together? How long would it be until we saw him again? Where was he now? Was he OK? Did he want to see us? Why did he leave?

Why did he leave? That was the most important question in my mind. I was totally confused. He wasn't there to answer our questions, so it was my mom who had to convince my sister and me that it wasn't our fault. My mom said all the right things, but none of them got through to me. It had happened, the reason for my forever box had finally come. My father wasn't dead but he was gone. I didn't know when we would see him or if I would see him. All I knew was that he was living in a hotel out by the airport. That was not enough to convince me that everything was going to be OK.

Everything was changing and I had lost all control. I had been so pompous, so sure, telling that girl at school that it couldn't happen to us. I cried every day and every night wondering why the separation had occurred, and for the loss of my father. I knew somehow, that it would never be the same between us. How could it be? Now I would be just like the girl at school seeing my dad once every other weekend, or at a restaurant over dinner; a Sunday father and child. I hadn't been able to get close to him before when he lived in our house so how could I do it now through an occasional visit?

My dad came back six weeks later. He was going to meet with my sister and me to explain why things had happened this way. He arrived unshaven and wrinkled, and I felt more sorry for him than I did for myself. He sat on the hearth of our fireplace, I sat in a rocking chair and my sister sat on the couch. We didn't hug each other or get close, we sat separately with our pain.

He tried to tell us why things were this way, but I was too upset to hear. It had been six weeks and my mind had already been made up. I believed that the reason why he left, at least in part, was because of me. I wasn't good enough, my grades weren't high enough, he didn't talk to me, I didn't make him happy. It was my fault. When you are failing at school and cannot seem to function in life without a spill or a noise, it is easy to feel that if something goes wrong it is your fault. Taking the blame was less complicated than trying to figure out why my mom had smiled through the pain and why I wasn't close enough to my dad to sense that he was unhappy. So there I was, with enough time to think about it and with very few answers except those I could come up with on my own. I thought that if I had been a perfect child, I could have made everything better for everyone.

CHAPTER
7

As I had suspected it would, everything changed after the divorce. My dad moved into an apartment building and my mom put our house up for sale. My mom, sister and I spent the summer clinging to each other to get through the pain. It was hard to see my mother crying or hurting because she had been the strong one all along. She was the one I knew best, and any weakness or sadness made me feel even more weak and vulnerable.

That summer went fast. We drove to California with another mother and daughter who were friends of ours. The trip was hard because it reminded us of the many trips that we had taken in our station wagon with my dad.

Those trips with my dad were fun. All of us in the car, my mom and dad in front and my sister and I with our toys and sleeping bags spread out in the back. My mom would bring a sack of little presents for us and if we remained quiet, every so often my mom would produce a surprise to reward us. The surprises were little dime store dolls or doll clothes. It didn't matter what it was, we looked forward to those surprises. My mom kept us busy and gave us something to look forward to on the long trips to California.

This trip was a little different. We were older now and the little bags of toys were no longer necessary. My mom drove the car this time. She was determined to drive the whole way just to prove that she could make it with or without my father. My dad had always been a quiet influence on these trips and in our life, so it wasn't his conversation that was missed, it was just having him there that we were used to.

The trip was as much fun as it could be under the circumstances. We went to Disneyland and Knott's Berry Farm. We laughed, but it was not the laughter of the years before. It was more hollow than that. The hardest part of the trip was that as much as we enjoyed the company of the mother and daughter whom we had brought along, every night they would call home to the father and brother who were waiting to hear from them. To listen to my young friend on the telephone say, "Oh, Daddy, I miss you and love you," made me feel terrible.

It seemed that the minute we left for the trip, we were looking forward to coming home. Getting away from our home didn't take away the reality of what life had become. My mom drove quickly on the way home. We dropped our two guests off at their house and they ran to the open arms of the family that was waiting. We went home to an empty house.

A NEW LIFE

We moved into a townhouse apartment about fifteen miles from our old neighborhood. It wasn't that far away, but we were in a new school district and had a new and different life. My mom was doing shows at one of the largest malls in the state, and we saw my dad once every other week at a restaurant or at his apartment.

Shawn and I would be attending a new school in the fall. I wasn't afraid; in fact, I thought that this would be a fresh start for me. A new school for some would mean leaving friends behind, but I didn't have many to leave. My third grade teacher was the only one I had been close to, and Billy and my other misfit friends had all gone away one at a time, either moving away from the neighborhood or to a different wing in the school. Going to a new school was actually a step forward.

As I thought about my new school, I made this little promise to myself that things would be different this year. I was going to be smart and I was going to have friends. I think I thought that if I was smart and popular, my parents would get back together and everything would be right again.

After we moved into our apartment, my sister and I spent most of our time in the pool at our complex. If we weren't in the pool, we were out meeting the kids who lived nearby. Most of the kids living in the apartments were from single parent families. They all seemed a little harder on the outside and a little wiser than we were. We were the new kids on the block. Divorce and all that it meant hadn't sunk in yet. We were fortunate enough to actually see our father and there hadn't been any custody battles, so we were not as advanced in the turmoils of life. The kids we met were a little rough around the edges, but they were kind to my sister and me.

My sister and I were changing. She was blossoming into a lovely lady and I was feeling like the title of a popular Judy Blume book, I Was a Ninety-Eight Pound Duckling. I had hips but no chest or shoulders, thick glasses and a forehead that was too big. I was thin as a rail and everyone was always trying to fatten me up. There would come a day when I would wish to be that thin again, but at the time, I felt scrawny and out of proportion.

That feeling of being an ugly duckling only grew worse as I saw my sister followed around by every boy she met. She didn't have to say or do anything, it was just the way she was. She was beautiful and smart and in seventh grade. I was a skinny fifth-grader who spent most of her time cleaning her room and dreaming of contact lenses.

The weather was beautiful that summer with daylight lasting until nine o'clock at night. On warm days we would swim until we were too tired to lift ourselves out of the pool. We would dry our hair, put on our jackets, and join the apartment kids in the bike park next to our complex.

We lived in a safe neighborhood. There was a police station, a bike park, a school, and a public swimming pool all within blocks of our apartment. I never worried that anything would happen to us while we were out playing in the neighborhood. Now that I am adult, I can imagine what it must have been like for my mother, worrying about our safety every minute of the day. Her work allowed her the flexibility to spend time with us, and she could take us to work with her if we weren't in school. But her fears never went away. She wanted to know where we were going at all times, and with whom. She was more protective now, maybe even too much so, but my sister and I knew that it was out of love.

My mother took good care of us. We knew that we could depend on her. But we also saw that she had her own pain to cope with. My mom recently told me that during that year there were times when she would ride a ferryboat while we were at school, then get home in time to meet us at the front door. She was adjusting to being alone, but the pain was so great that she would sit on a ferryboat and let the waves soothe the hurt.

I know that in many ways my mom felt that she had failed. Women in her generation had been brought up to be good little housewives and mothers. The marriage had failed for a lot of reasons and still she held to those old fashioned values of, "If it fell apart, it must have been my fault."

She did stand by my dad long after the marriage had crumbled. Even when it fell apart, she still held on to what it used to be. She would express some anger about Dad around us, but she never kept us from seeing him. It is a credit to both my parents that there never was a custody battle or wars in court over my sister and me. My dad knew that we would be better off with my mom and he never pushed the issue.

After the sixties, you might think that my mom was a real liberated woman, but she wasn't. She was liberated in business and could live on her own and support us. She could do all those things, but she later told me that somehow she felt that whether or not the marriage was working, having any man there was better than not having one at all. She felt as some women still do today, that they aren't as good without the approval of a man.

My mom was supporting us and paying bills even when my dad was still with us. So why the insecurity? First of all, it was how she was raised. A family of four, with a dad who participated, a mother who was strong and a marriage still intact. The family held together through thick and thin. I realize the failure that she must have felt for having a marriage that fell apart. It happens so often now we are not surprised, but back then, divorce was something that only happened to other people.

If she had been the one to leave, it would have been different, and her insecurities wouldn't have been so great. But he left her. No matter how much she tried to convince herself that she was still a worthwhile person, in the back of her mind she wondered why she wasn't good enough. And wondered, "If I had been smarter, more clever and more loving, would I have been able to hold this marriage together?"

That summer, we became "just the three of us." It was quite an adjustment. We each hurt in our own way, but none of us were completely alone. We had each other. We would snuggle together in my mom's room whenever the loneliness set in. Time would make things better, but during those first nights alone in our apartment, it seemed that life would always feel this way.

FIFTH GRADE

When school started, I was prepared. My mom gave my sister and I fifty dollars each to buy new school clothes. It doesn't sound like much according to today's standards, but when I was in fifth grade, it seemed like all the money in the world. I worked hard to look for the sales so that I could get as many clothes with my fifty dollars as was humanly possible.

Once I had the clothes, then I had to have the right glasses. This particular year wire framed glasses were in style, and I wanted them very badly. The only problem was that my lenses were thick and the wire frames were thin. That meant that every time I tripped or someone patted me on the back, my lenses popped out. I spent the entire next year popping my lenses back into the frames every time they fell out.

Now I had the clothes and glasses, I just needed the right folders, pencils, and pencil boxes. We went to a big drugstore that was having a huge back-to-school sale. I stocked up on every folder, ruler, notebook, and school supply that I could find. Somehow I thought that the more folders I had, the larger my pencil boxes were, the smarter I would be. I wish it were that simple.

I walked into school the first day with my thick glasses and my stack of notebooks and everyone thought I was really smart. Now that's a change!

I prepared for that first day so intensely because I knew that this was my big chance. No one knew me at this school. Nobody knew whether I was smart or not, and I wasn't about to tell them about my problems. I wasn't going to tell the teacher, either. My mom and I had learned that it was best not to say anything about my learning disabilities unless it was absolutely necessary. It seemed that the less people knew, the better off I was.

I knew that I would probably have some learning problems that year. I had come to accept this. But there was something different about being at a new school where I had a new identity and a new start. I really felt relieved that the old school and early assessments were far enough behind me that I could go on.

The school that I would be attending was just across the bike park from our townhouse. I could walk through the complex, through the bike park, and in ten minutes I was at school. It was a small school with only one teacher and one classroom per grade level. I was put into the only fifth grade classroom that they had, Mr. Peters' class. I knew very early that it was going to be a rough year.

This school was extremely small. If there was a resource room, I never knew about it. Those of us who sat in the lowest reading group and got the lowest scores on our tests would have liked extra help. We never did get it. When I didn't receive any help for my problems in class, I assumed that the school must not have read my file. Or maybe they never got my file in the first place. If they had, why didn't I get any help?

After that first move, I got the impression that maybe school officials didn't analyze the new kids' files as I had imagined. Maybe there wasn't the time or the energy to do so. It relieved me to know that maybe they didn't know as much about my past as I thought. As much as I needed help, it made me feel better to know that I wasn't labeled before I ever got started.

MR. PETERS

Mr. Peters was close to retirement and sick of kids. He was raised in the old school of parenting that said that all kids should be seen and not heard, and in the old school of teaching that said that all kids can be taught in the same way and will progress at the same level. If only life were that cut and dried.

He read futuristic science fiction books and melancholy stories when he read aloud to us. I hated those stories, but he thrived on them. That might give you an idea of what his personality was like.

There were times when I saw a side of him that was really nice. On a good day he even had a little sense of humor, but most of the time I got the feeling that he would lose his mind if one more kid asked another question. Whenever he got mad at us he would shake his finger and say, "You kids nowadays have no respect for authority," or "You kids nowadays are spoiled, you have just been handed everything." He often sounded like the comedic lines made famous by Bill Cosby, "When I was a kid, we didn't have anything. I had to walk fifty miles to school, in the snow, barefoot! In fact when I was a boy, we didn't even have air!"

He taught school during the day and managed an old movie theater at night. I think I was the only student in our class who knew this. I happened to go to the movie theater one night and saw him there. When I went up to say hello, he told me and my mom that he was the manager and he took me on a tour of the theater. It was a beautiful place and Mr. Peters seemed a lot nicer in this different atmosphere than he ever was in the classroom.

READING GROUPS

Within a few weeks, the class was separated into reading groups; I was put into the lowest group. Each group would be called up one at a time. While the other kids in the class read silently, our group, the lowest one, was always called up last. I hated being labeled low, medium, and high; and I hated the fact that everyone was reading silently while we fumbled through our easy reading books.

This was exactly how we were separated in the first grade. Even though the circle that we sat in was back several feet from the rest of the class, you were sure that they could hear you sounding out each word and listening as the teacher corrected you. Whether I was five or eleven, I felt the peer pressure and worried about being different.

I can remember sitting in that circle, book in hand, my teacher looking at the group while most of us looked at the floor. The first child would start with her halting reading and around the circle we would go. I hated starting first but at least I got it over with. When I was last in line it felt like I was waiting for punishment. I would get a knot in my stomach as the teacher signaled me to read, and I lifted my book with dread.

My old habits were still there. I still tended to follow a sentence with my head rather than with my eyes. My head would move from side to side as I read. My teacher would then correct me and say that we were to track a sentence with our eyes, not our head. I would try to hold my head still, but my eyes would not stay on one line. They went all over. My teacher also tried to break me of the habit of using my finger, a bookmark or a piece of paper to keep my eyes on the right line. My finger acted as a guide for my eyes and a paper or bookmark helped me to block out the other distractions on the page. Everything from a picture to the other words on the page could distract me, so I learned as time went on to block out the extra distractions and keep the focus on what I needed.

My teacher didn't allow this. The bookmarks and paper were taken away, and it was absolutely out of the question to follow with your finger. He had been taught to not let us use our finger to guide our eyes along. For most kids, that was probably a good rule. Other kids, in time, would learn to track with their eyes, and using their finger was just a crutch. But I was not like most kids. I took away my finger and found myself struggling to stay on track and focus again.

I found myself very frustrated with school because I was expected to learn in the same way that everyone else was learning. I felt the expectation to conform with the group and I tried never to stray from the norm. As long as I continued to try to learn just like everyone else, I never really succeeded beyond the below average or average level academically.

WHEN IT GETS TOO TOUGH TO STAY SILENT

I said earlier that my mom and I had learned that the best way to deal with my learning problems was not to make a big issue of them, unless it became a problem that we could no longer avoid. I knew that I was harder to teach, so I expected a few hassles or misunderstandings. I'm not saying that being embarrassed or yelled at is not devastating; it is. I came home so many times and cried to myself and to my mom about a hurtful remark or action that had taken place at school. I could have had a conference every time something came up, but I didn't want people to know more than they had to about my learning problems.

I am sure that there are a lot of people who would have handled it differently than we did. They would have gone in on the first day of school for teacher conferences to explain their situation. I know that we could have chosen to tell people right away about my problems. I don't believe that would have helped, especially when I was in school. They had names for some of my problems, but they didn't have any answers. In truth, there were many teachers who didn't even know what dyslexia was. Young teachers just out of school might, but not teachers like the one I had in fifth grade. Mention the word "disability" and everyone starts saying, "Not in my room." People get worried when you mention a word that might mean more work, and more hardship for them. I don't really blame them, but I still needed their help.

When things just got too tough to continue on in silence, my mother usually had to go to school. I hated this part of my learning problems because you never knew what could happen. Fortunately, my mom could politely tell someone that there was a problem without making them feel defensive. This is a hard thing to do. If you don't put something the right way, people feel pushed and put down. Their usual response when under fire is to fight back. If my mom had handled it the wrong way, she could have ended up making matters worse for me.

The first time that I came home crying from my fifth grade class was after we had just taken our first math test. When the test had been corrected and the teacher was handing them out, he didn't just hand them out, he listed the scores on the board so that everyone could see how the other people had done. I was humiliated. My name was written last on the list, with the lowest score, and now the whole class knew. I felt everyone looking at me. My face was hot with embarrassment. I sat through the rest of the day and refused to let the kids see me cry.

As soon as my mom came home, I told her about the whole ordeal. She wanted to go talk to my teacher, but I begged her not to. It was only about the third week of school and I didn't want to start something so early in the year. I decided to give it a little time to see if the situation changed. My mom agreed not to talk to Mr. Peters in person but instead, she wrote a letter. I brought it to school and gave it to him. He took the letter and threw it in the bottom drawer of his desk. I don't believe that he ever read it.

Things didn't get better, but they didn't get worse. Fortunately, I had my mom to talk to if I needed a sympathetic shoulder.

A few months into the year, it was time for something to be done. My teacher was growing more and more impatient with me. There were many things about me that annoyed him, but my asking questions all the time bothered him the most.

One day, I was at his desk several times to ask questions. This was not unusual; in one day I was in and out of my seat much more than any other student. Because it took repetition for me to learn, I needed to hear the answer to my question more than once. On this particular day, I had gone up to his desk to ask a question one too many times. On the final trip, he just started yelling. He yelled, "Shari, stop coming up to my desk all the time. You go sit down. You are not the only person in this class. You take up more time than anyone else. Go sit down. Go sit down!"

The whole class got quiet for a minute. I sat down in humiliation. It was at a time like this that I could turn to no one. I wanted to cry but I held it in. When a break came, I went in the bathroom and let the tears go.

I hid my pain until I got home and could talk to my mom. When I told her, she decided to go to school and meet with my teacher.

My mom said that my teacher nodded his head and listened to what she had to say. He listened, but nothing changed after that. He never fully accepted me. But he also didn't yell at me again, he just ignored me.

Every time a problem arose with a teacher, or any authority figure for that matter, I felt more and more powerless. Powerless to learn, powerless to fit into the world and to meet the expectations that surrounded me.

I was full of anger and frustration but had no place to go with it. I couldn't get mad at my teacher; I was taught to be a good little girl. Good little girls don't make big noises, yell, or fight back. Instead of putting the anger in its proper place, I internalized it. When people were mean to me, I was mad at myself, not them. Their anger and rejection fueled me into trying to please them and make myself better according to their standards.

Needing my father's attention and praise, and never getting any of it, made me needy in all areas of my life. I needed more from my teachers and more from my friends. I was constantly in need of love and praise. When I didn't get it, or even worse, when I was hurt by someone important to me, I was emotionally crushed.

I often think that it was my needs that pushed people away. I needed a lot of love and my dad didn't know how to give it to me, so I felt that he didn't love me at all. I wanted to be liked by the teachers, so I would try hard and ask a lot of questions, trying desperately to keep up. My intensity and my hidden challenges tended to make people afraid and uncomfortable, so they avoided me. Yet it was me who needed their acceptance most.

WHERE DO YOU GO WITH THE FRUSTRATION?

I had learned to cover my emotions so that I wouldn't bother people more than I already did, but these emotions burned a hole inside of me. Some kids channel that same emotion by becoming rebellious or cynical and by displaying behavioral problems in the classroom. Neither are great options. Holding the emotion in makes you helpless and afraid. Letting the emotion out repels people away at a time when you most need people to love and care about you.

I know that just as children and young adults get angry at themselves and their situations, so do parents. As a parent, but especially as the parent of a child with challenges, there is an automatic reaction to lash out at those who hurt your child. It was to my benefit that my mom was able to tactfully handle those who didn't understand me. She knew that she had to take a deep breath before she went into a conference. If she didn't, she probably would say something that put the person that she was dealing with on the defensive, which in the long run wouldn't help me.

I think that it is important for parents to know that it is all right to get angry and want to get back at those who hurt your child. But when you shove, people automatically want to shove back. If you go in with your fists waving, it could drastically affect your chances of working with that teacher in an effective way. I think there are always circumstances that require a "get tough" attitude, but at the same time, you have to think about the effect of your actions in the long run. Be tough but walk lightly. Praise while asking for changes.

Regarding your children, it is important to teach them to speak up for themselves in a positive and articulate way. To speak on behalf of themselves they must know what their disabilities are and how to explain them even in the simplest form at a very early age.

If you always speak for them, they will always be helpless. If you teach them to explain their problems and ask for help in a positive way rather than acting out, being destructive, or not doing anything at all, they will be on their way to surviving in the world. If they know their differences, they can make changes and help others to help them. If they have to wait for someone to rescue them, they will be walking invalids. What will they do if you aren't there? Teach them to take over the battle and to fight it in a positive way.

School did not get any easier during fifth grade, but one thing did change that year. I had friends, true friends, for the first time in my life.

I met these friends in a way that was unusual for me. I didn't beg them to like me, they came to me. I didn't have to make fun of myself to entertain them. I didn't have to buy them things or compromise myself to get them to like me. They just liked me. Aside from a few precious others, these friendships were the best that I have ever known.

Amy, Katie, and Heidi were not from divorced families, and they didn't have learning problems. They were so normal that I couldn't believe it when they came up and talked to me. I was used to attracting the misfits of life and protecting the underdogs in a crisis. Now, here were these three girls who could be friends with anyone, and they wanted to be friends with me.

What a great feeling it was to come to school and know that my math score wasn't important to them. My life's history didn't matter, I did. It was so great, so equal. I could just be myself and that was enough. I had seldom experienced that kind of acceptance. I know now that my three friends thought of me as just that - a friend. There wasn't a sign on my head that said "reject" or any of the other names I'd been called; it was just how I felt about myself that made me feel others wouldn't accept me.

Every recess was spent out on the jungle gym, our skinny legs hanging through the open spaces. We would spend that time telling stories and jokes, gossiping and talking about our more than eccentric teacher. It was such fun laughing and talking, not being on guard or worried about saying something wrong. I was just one of the girls.

Fond memories of that year were because of those three girls. I even joined the Blue Birds to be with them! Blue Birds were required to sell mints, and I hated that. I always came up short on my mint money. But even worse was that Blue Birds had to wear blue polyester pants and a blue felt vest for every Tuesday afternoon meeting. But to be with my friends, I would even wear blue polyester pants and sell candy.

I still keep in touch with all three of them. We only see each other once a year or so, but the friendship is still strong. They are the only friends that I have from any early grade, which says how special they are to me.

I know that they didn't see me as a weird kid or a learning disabled kid. In fact, I can remember telling Heidi's mom, when I was eighteen, that I wanted to write a book about my learning problems. She couldn't believe it. "You have learning problems?!" It wasn't a topic of conversation that I liked to bring up when I was in fifth grade. I struggled, and continued to struggle, but didn't talk a lot about it. I was Amy's, Katie's, and Heidi's friend; and whether they knew about them or not, they didn't seem to care about my differences.

THE LIBRARY

Friends come in many different forms. Mrs. Sager, my mom, and my third grade teacher were friends. Most of the time I couldn't relate to people my own age, or should I say, they couldn't relate to me; so I gravitated toward whoever cared about me. Age was not a factor, just love, acceptance, and friendship. Yes, there were times I wished I had more friends my own age that were acceptable and popular, but the love of an adult could so often make up for what I didn't get from children my own age.

In fifth grade, I was lucky enough to have Amy, Katie, and Heidi. But I also, just by chance, met a wonderful friend who, probably unknowingly, touched my life. She was the librarian at our school and I was in the lowest reading group in my fifth grade class. Not a likely pair, but we got along all the same.

For most of my fifth grade year, I walked to school alone. I enjoyed that quiet time. It was that time before the noise of a classroom filled with kids invaded my jumbled mind. I didn't mind being alone or in silence, that was my time to sort things out and get in control. The fifteen minute walk was my preparation for a scattered day, that would be spent facing my learning problems.

My mom was working during my fifth grade year, and when she left for work I didn't like to stay in the house alone. So I would leave early and wander around the school until our classroom opened. I was used to planning ahead for my possible mistakes

113

and any changes in routine that I might have to endure in the morning, so I was always up earlier than necessary. I had an extra fifteen to thirty minutes each morning just in case I forgot something or didn't lock the front door and had to go back.

Other people would have relished the extra half hour of sleep, but I used it to help me follow up on what my brain missed in the morning. To me, the extra sleep wasn't worth sitting in class all day wondering if I had left the iron on. The way my brain worked, if I didn't check and recheck it, I wasn't sure that I had done it.

Once I checked everything around the house, I would leave for school early. I felt more prepared arriving at school early rather than late and hurried. I knew my limits and being hurried only caused me problems. However, once at school, there was no place for me to go and nothing for me to do.

When it rained, I would often stand underneath the overhang by the library. Every day I would see the librarian, who also arrived early, preparing the library for a busy day.

The rule was that nobody was supposed to be in the library before the first bell rang. That was the librarian's preparation time and she needed it without kids standing around and moving things. I didn't know this rule when I first started going to school.

There were many cold mornings when I went to school and stood outside the library, hoping the librarian would take pity on me and let me in. I soon figured out the rules when she pointed at the clock and mouthed the message through the window that she couldn't let me in until the first bell.

I was persistent, you have to give me that. I kept coming to school and standing outside the library shivering in the cold. That poor librarian said the same thing everyday, "I can't let you in until the first bell." When the cold Seattle winter rains began to fall, I stood even closer to the library door. There wasn't anything she could do to avoid seeing me, and finally she just let me come in.

At first she was quiet and didn't really say anything. She just let me come in, get warm, and do some of my homework at one of the tables. Gradually, we got to know each other a little bit. We only made small talk, but it was so nice to have an adult friend at that school.

I felt privileged that she let me come into the library early, and she even let me help her sort books once in a while. She didn't have to be nice to me or talk to me, but she was very kind. She even saved books for me about my most loved of all subjects, horses.

I was very lucky to have come into contact with people like her from time to time. I don't think we give enough recognition to all the people who work in a school. It isn't just the teachers who have an impact on kids, it's anyone the kids come in contact with from morning to night. Anyone can touch children's lives and help them to feel good about themselves - secretaries, librarians, janitors, cooks, and bus drivers. The people who put feeling and love into their jobs will reach students, no matter what their position.

I had a janitor make a comment to me which ended with, "But then again, I'm just the janitor." If all you are is "just a janitor," how can you be an integral part of making that school run and making a difference in kids' lives? I'm glad that my librarian friend didn't just look at her job as being "just the librarian" or look at the rule, "No kids in the library before the first bell," as absolute. She was a quiet, but kind, influence on me. She made me feel important by saving books for me, and by letting me help her around the library. A few kind words, and I would have helped her do anything. She was not "just the librarian" to me.

HORSES

My librarian friend found a way to reach me through reading that even I hadn't found before - books on horses. Every book on that subject that she could find, she saved for me. Up to that point, I had seldom picked up a book to read for leisure. Even though I was able to read, I avoided it because I struggled with it so much. There was so much reading required for school that it took up most of my time. She changed that!

My love for horses never died. But my dream of having a horse in my backyard was fading. We didn't even have a backyard; where would you put a horse in an apartment? My dream was moving farther and farther away from reality but it was still worth having. Dreaming about horses was good for me. It was something positive to think about when things weren't going right. It was like singing. When I was singing, I was somebody and it helped me cope with life. Dreaming about horses and the occasional contact that I had with them gave me the goal to be a good rider and to someday own a horse.

I had only had a few opportunities to ride a horse, but each time I did have the chance I found myself feeling natural and in control, more in control than in any other circumstance. I wasn't afraid or even nervous. It came naturally and whatever I didn't know, I could learn about by watching people and reading books.

THE PASTURE

Before my parents' divorce we had lived in a house that was on a fairly busy street and a very steep hill. It would not have

115

been safe for me to walk alone on that street or in the immediate vicinity.

Now we were living in a quiet neighborhood with a police station and school nearby. I seldom spent time after school over at friends' houses. With my mom working and my sister at her friends' houses or at after school activities, it meant I had some extra hours to myself in the afternoon.

When early spring came and the weather improved, I began looking around beyond our apartment complex, even beyond the bike park or my schoolyard. This was risky considering I have very little sense of direction. I might go somewhere many times, but I won't recognize the area when I see it again, or I'll get it confused with another area that looks similar.

Though most fifth graders have an extensive "mental map" of their neighborhoods, I never knew what was beyond my own front porch unless I had been there many times and had been forced to find my way back on my own. If I could find my way there and back, even if it was by trial and error, it was usually ingrained in my memory. Until several months after moving in, I didn't even know that our apartment complex went around in a circle of buildings. I would go for walks, but I was too scared to go beyond the pool and cabana area because I didn't know if I could find my way back. I couldn't believe it when I found out that the complex was just a few buildings arranged in a circle and not some big complex where I could get lost.

Once I got the nerve, I ventured past my well known territory of the school yard and the apartment complex, and I found what I thought was a dream. A horse pasture with horses everywhere. Here I was the horse lover of the century, and I found a horse pasture practically at my backdoor.

I started spending every afternoon there watching the horses, and occasionally, a rider who was exercising a horse. I came to love these peaceful times sitting on the fence, watching those wonderful animals that I had only rarely been able to get close to.

At some point during the school year, my friend Heidi told me that she had a horse at the local pasture. Little did I know that she actually had five (several were Arabians) and that she and her sisters had been showing horses for years.

I looked up to Heidi and I felt bonded with her because she shared my love of horses. It was because of her and her sisters that I learned how to ride. Even when I moved away, she and her family always invited me to come over and stay with them, which meant going to the pasture and seeing the horses. With each visit I became a better rider, and for those few moments up on that horse I was in command and felt like somebody.

116

When we moved, it was Amy, Katie, Heidi, the librarian, and the peaceful afternoons I spent at the pasture that I missed the most.

WEEKEND FATHER AND DAUGHTER

Even with the positive aspects of my fifth grade year, I was still working hard to deal with being the kid of a divorced family. The dinners every other week and the once in a while overnight stays were exactly what I had feared. I didn't know my father before, and now I had even less time to get to know him.

Time was a barrier. How much can you learn about a kid who is already eleven and growing fast if there is no time? Before, it was my Dad's work and now it was two separate households that divided us. I still desperately needed my father's attention. The separation and lack of time with him only made me want him more.

We shared small talk at those dinners out or during the weekends at his apartment. I had so much I wanted to say to him, but I felt that my dad wasn't comfortable with me or my feelings. I felt that I had to be a happy kid and say everything was fine - hide the emotions because it is less messy. Maybe that isn't what my dad intended. Or maybe he could just file his emotions away or handle them in private. I couldn't, but to please him I tried.

My dad would come to pick us up once every other week to take us out for pizza or to a Mexican restaurant for dinner. I used to think that I was a pretty lucky kid because I thought that I probably went out to dinner more than most kids. Having pizza every other week is the best thing I can say about divorce.

It became common for me to sit across the table from my sister and my dad. It wasn't planned, it just kind of worked out that way. They sat across from me and, since I was different, it seemed right somehow.

My sister had a lot of things to talk about. She had school and good grades. I, on the other hand, would stray towards horses and Blue Birds. I can't say that the conversation often fell to me. The most that I can remember anybody ever saying to me was, "Don't order what you won't eat, Shari."

I just sat there and, for the most part, hoped that the conversation would not require me to talk. What would I talk about? School? Emotions? No, we were in a restaurant for goodness sake. So what did I say? Very little.

I would stare at my food and keep myself very busy so that I wouldn't open my mouth and say something wrong. I tried to talk sometimes, but nothing ever came out right and I ended up regretting that I had said anything at all.

Then there were those times when we spent the night at my dad's apartment. Those were always kind of stiff times. Once again, I couldn't be myself because when I was myself, I was usually spilling, laughing, or getting in the way. It was a small place for a kid like me so I tried to stay in control and be quiet.

Everything was in order at my dad's house. Everything was always in order in my room, but it was my order and my room. If I messed something up, I could always put it back. At my dad's, I was so worried about messing something up or breaking something that I found myself sitting on the corner of the couch with my glass of 7-Up and a dish of peanuts in front of me, afraid to move.

My dad wouldn't have yelled if I spilled something. But I was so worried about disappointing him in the little time that we had together, I sat on pins and needles trying not to do anything wrong. I was so self-conscious, he would have had to hug me a million times to reassure me that he wasn't going to go away or hate me if I spilled my 7-Up or dropped a peanut. I felt bad about myself and thought that I was responsible for my parents' divorce. That was a pretty heavy load on a fifth grader's shoulders. Maybe if my dad had talked more, I would have known how he really felt about me; but he would have had to tell me many times to make me believe I was not a mess in his eyes.

When I spoke about things I wanted to do or liked to do, Dad often said, "You're just like your mother." Maybe he didn't intend for it to be hurtful, but as a kid I could only take it in one way. In my mind I answered with, "You left my mother because you stopped loving her. You say I'm like her, so maybe you'll leave me, too."

It was just a passing, off-hand comment made over dinner. "You're just like your mother." When he said this, it burned me inside because it reinforced that need to please and to be better so that he wouldn't leave me.

As a result of not wanting to have my dad say I was like my mom, I stopped almost all productions and entertainment by fifth grade. I stopped doing those things for several years thinking that it would prevent my father from ever leaving me.

I was a kid searching, grasping for pieces that would help the puzzle make sense. It wouldn't make sense for a long time. My father thought I knew he loved me, and I continued to run after him, begging for his attention.

CONTROL/CLEANING

As time went on, I felt that I had little or no control over my world. As an eleven year old, I couldn't stop people from doing

118

what they wanted. I knew that I couldn't keep divorce from happening, or control what my teacher thought of me. But in my own way, I gained control in the only place where I could, my room.

In our first house, I had begun my ritual of cleaning anything and everything around the house. The only thing that I did daily was clean my room. From early on, my room was in impeccable shape and neat as a pin.

When we moved to the apartment, the same was true. My room was still in order but now even more so. More than that, at some point early in the year, I took over the position of resident house cleaner. I would clean the whole house top to bottom everyday. I had an apron, scrub brushes, and rubber gloves.

When I came home from school, I didn't do my homework first. I cleaned the house. I scrubbed the showers, cleaned the toilets, and even did the laundry. No one was home when I got home and only occasionally did my sister not have after school plans, so the house was mine.

The funny thing was that nobody was making me do this. I liked cleaning. It was like therapy for me. The harder or more upsetting the day, the more cleaning I would do. Cleaning somehow put my mind at ease. I went through my routines without thinking; I already knew what to do and I did it well.

When I started cleaning, the house was a mess and in disarray, just like my brain felt. When I had cleaned the house and all it's contents were in order, my brain felt like it was in order, too. Cleaning put everything where it belonged and it uncovered what I couldn't find. It also kept me in touch with where my things were since my mind had such a short memory.

The therapeutic value was that it required no talking or intense mental energy from me, I just did it. When I was done, I felt peaceful and could go on to my homework. When I first came home from a scattered day at school, my mind was too jumbled to start school work. Cleaning calmed me, settled me and helped me get out all of my extra energy so that I could concentrate and sit still. It helped reduce anger and frustration because I was moving, scrubbing, bending, and puffing around the house and up and down the stairs. If I was frustrated, I would take it out on the house by scrubbing.

I still find cleaning to be one of the best ways to clear my mind and put order to a mixed up day. If I am upset about something, look out - the house will be immaculate! It still works for me today.

I know at some point that my cleaning may have gone to an extreme. Maybe I was too orderly and yet, in many ways, it was that order that helped me to survive. I told you earlier that organization skills are what help a learning disabled person survive;

in my own way I was learning to deal with my learning problems by cleaning and developing organizational skills. I just hadn't learned how to apply these skills to school.

I cleaned the only domain that I had. Outside my front door I may have felt out of control, but in my house I had the control to put things right and to get rid of the dust and the dirt. When I removed that dirt or took out the garbage, it was like throwing out the bad news and happenings of the day. I would sweep the floor of its dirt and in some way it also swept my mind of its problems.

At some point it came to be that clean was not clean enough, organized was not organized enough, perfect was not perfect enough. It was my control and my vent for frustration. My cleaning rituals were for me what work is to the workaholic, food or lack of it to an anorexic, or any other compulsive behavior. I was repeating one behavior to mask a whole set of feelings.

Why? For all my life I had been the mess-up, the out of control child. I found a way to feel more perfect and to get in control. Get rid of the dirt from the counter and somehow it takes the dirt out of your life; organize your books and papers and for that moment you feel better about the fact that you can't read the book or write the essay.

Washing my hands, as with cleaning, was done in repetition as if I thought I was dirty. Washing my hands until my skin was so dry that I bled was my way of making the imperfect side of me go away. To me it was order, control, and a release. I guess maybe I thought that if I washed long enough and hard enough, I wouldn't be bad anymore.

Why do people starve themselves to have attention and love? I can't say that my route was so different, just less destructive. I was grabbing onto something that I could control.

People find all kinds of ways to cope - drinking, smoking, eating, excessive sleeping; I chose cleaning. What mother wouldn't hope that her children learn how to deal with their problems as I did? My mom didn't mind my cleaning, but she was very worried about my blood stained hands. Eventually I stopped washing my hands excessively, but cleaning continued to bring me peace in some strange way.

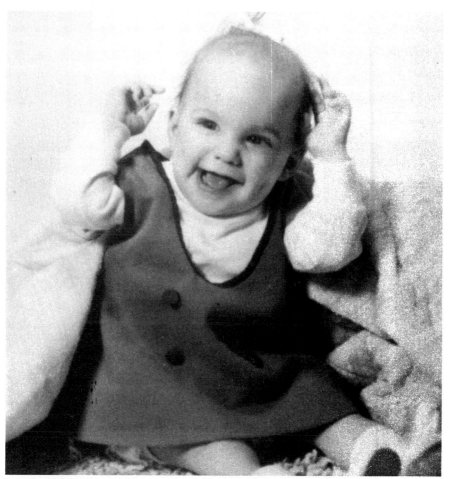

3 months old. Someone was holding me up from behind in this picture — amazing, I'm not crying.

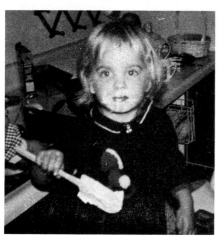

18 months old. I am not having a good day!

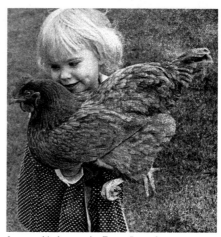

2 years old. Are you the Easter Bunny?

I

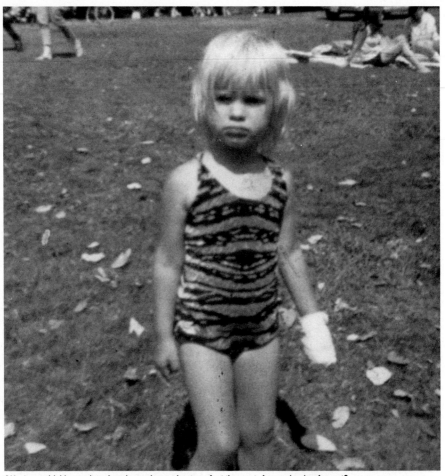

2½ years old. I burned my hand one day and cut my foot the next. Are we having fun yet?

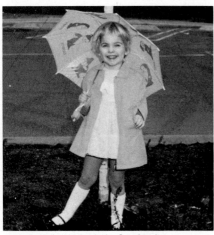

4 years old. I'm singing in the Seattle rain.

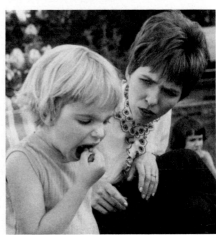

3 years old. Ready to eat anything, even when Mom says no.

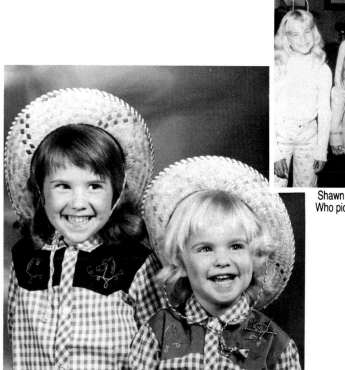

Shawn and I at ages 9 and 11.
Who picked out these clothes?

My sister Shawn and I at 2 and 4 years old.
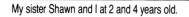

Shawn and I at 18
and 20 at a college function.

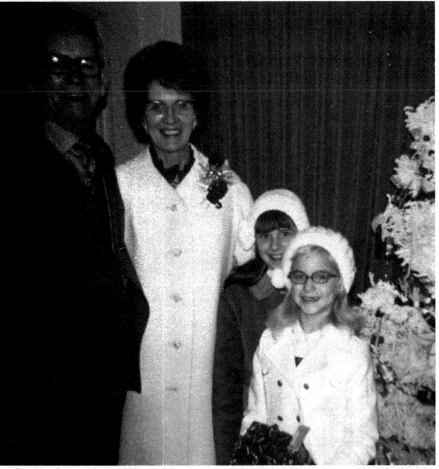

My Grandma, Grandpa, Shawn and I at Christmas.

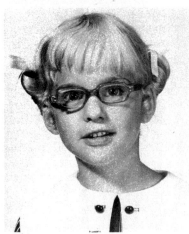

My kindergarten school picture. I'm either Buffy from "Family Affair" or Princess Lea from "Star Wars".

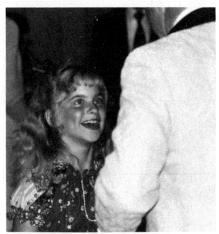

I was in second grade here. This was one of the few pictures in which I thought I looked pretty.

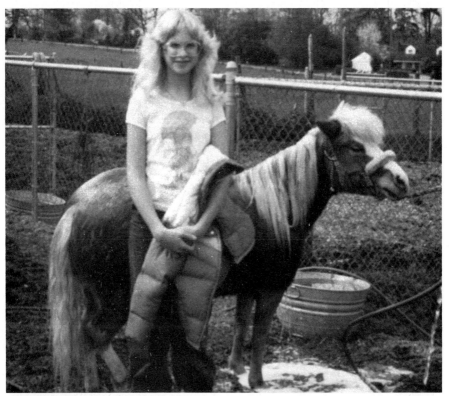

Me, a pony named Misty and my blue tinted glasses during my sixth grade year.

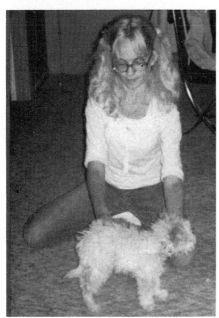

Scotty and I, and a pair of brown glasses, during the summer before my 6th grade year.

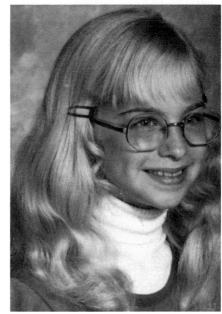

A must for fifth grade — wire framed glasses.

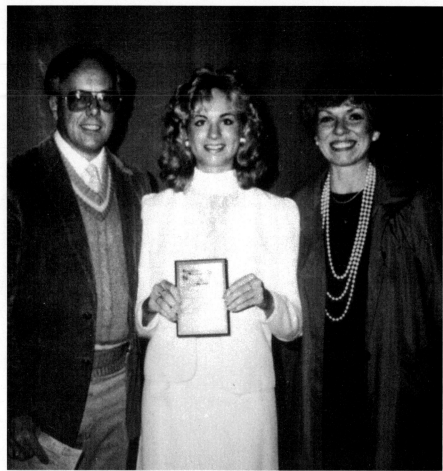

My Mom, stepdad, and me at my senior awards assembly. I am holding the ASB (Associated Student Body) award.

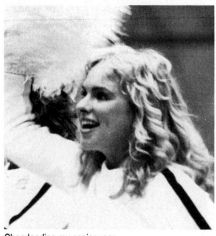

Cheerleading my senior year.

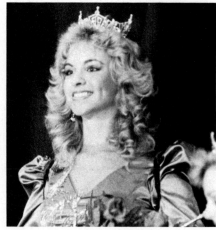

Winning a local pageant — beginning my speaking career.

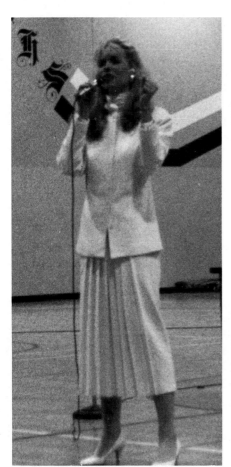

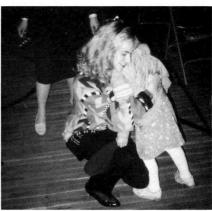

Hugging a child after an assembly at an elementary school.

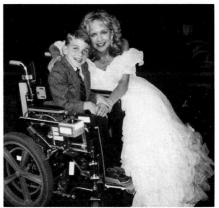

It looks so simple in this picture. I'm actually looking at 2000 students at this moment.

A friend and I taking publicity photos for my first book.

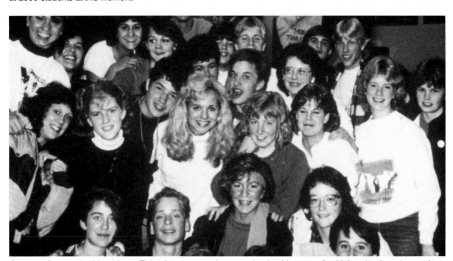

Can you find me in this picture. This picture was taken at a leadership camp for high school students where I was a presenter.

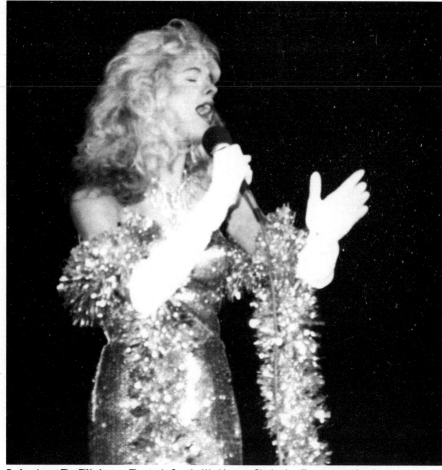

Performing at The Fifth Avenue Theater in Seattle, Washington. Singing is still my greatest love!

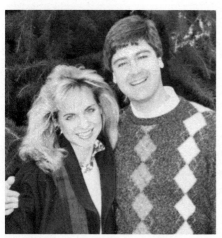

I take that back — David is my greatest love.

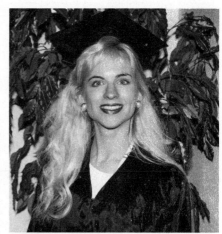

Graduation Day! University of Washington.

CHAPTER
8

NEW MEN IN MY LIFE

My fifth grade year brought many changes, divorce, a new school; and then came the biggest change of all, my parents started dating. I never wanted my parents to split up and now I am supposed to let another person like them - and me. No way! My mom said, "Be nice," and I tried to be, but it is a "twilight zone" feeling when your dad says he is going to take you and your sister out to dinner and asks if we mind if he brings a friend? What friend? Bill, the car salesman friend? No, Nancy, the receptionist friend. It's a weird feeling when you are in fifth grade and your parents are single.

My mom only dated a couple of people after the divorce. One of the men that she dated was Bob, and it seemed that once she met him, she stopped dating anyone else. "He is a family man," she said, "who has two kids of his own." Maybe because he had two kids and one of the two lived with him, it made her feel secure and think that he was interested in the same thing that she was - family.

I think, looking back, my mom would agree that she jumped into a serious relationship far too soon. Her reason? Being a single mother was not easy, the loneliness of being single, or the feelings that to be whole again would only come by being married, were all the reasons that she needed. Financially we were surviving, and emotionally we had each other to lean on. But I think my mom isolated herself and looked for a commitment so soon because she wanted us to be a whole family again.

My mom stopped taking other invitations for dates and waited by the phone for Bob to call. I really didn't know him so I wasn't concerned that she was seeing only him, nor did it occur to me that any relationship would turn into a marriage less than a year after my parents' divorce.

The first time that I met Bob was when I joined him and my mom on one of their dates. It was a very quiet meeting. I think Bob and I may have said two words to each other the whole night. When we came back home my mom said, "Isn't he a great person?" I agreed, to please her; but to tell you the truth, I didn't know him, and I wasn't sure that I wanted to know him.

Months passed and Bob remained the only person in Mom's life. My sister and I didn't really get involved with it until my mom announced that they were going to get married. Marriage was the furthest thing from our minds. We were just getting settled and fitting into our new life.

If it had been a great idea, my sister and I wouldn't have said anything. I mean that truthfully. If I had felt that my mom and Bob's marriage would last and that she had really found her match, I would have been happy for them. Instead, my sister and I were terrified. We told my mom of our concerns, but she couldn't hear us clearly at the time.

I went into a lot of reasons why I knew it wasn't going to work out, and my sister did as well. Later, my mom admitted that she also saw signs of turbulence before they were married. But just like the marriage to my father, regardless of problems, she was determined to make things work. My mom put on her winning smile, as she always did; and for a while, she even had me convinced that Bob was a great guy and that everything was going to be wonderful. She could do that - make you think everything was just fine. What she couldn't do was make us love Bob.

My sister made it clear from the start that she would have little to do with him. She would tolerate him and his kids, but nothing more. I admired her strength. The way she was able to handle it turned out to be the best way in our circumstance. If she didn't get too attached, nothing would be lost if it didn't work out.

I too wanted to fight all of these changes being thrown my way. A marriage, another move, a stepfather, and a new brother and sister. But I was not strong enough to protest. All of the fight had been drained out of me when I learned that to be accepted both in and out of the classroom, I must be good and never cause a disruption. I was afraid, but I kept my feelings hidden so I wouldn't disappoint anyone, especially my mom. To please everyone around me, I dove in and tried to like, and even love, the new members of our family.

I felt torn. On one hand, I wanted to have the perfect family situation. Sometimes I even tried to believe that is what we had. But it was all just a fantasy. This new family was doomed from the start and I found myself wishing I had never formed any attachment at all with Bob or his children.

SAYING GOOD-BYE

I can remember as the end of my fifth grade year approached, I learned more and more about the plans for that summer. When my sister and I were out of school, we would pack up and move to an apartment in the city near where Bob lived. Bob and my mom would get married before school started and then we would move into Bob's house.

I can remember feeling that, for the first time, I actually had someone to say good-bye to. During our first move, I said good-bye to people, but I never feared not seeing them again. I did fear never seeing Amy, Katie, and Heidi again. My first real friends were going to be left behind.

One day out on the playground, Amy, Katie, Heidi, and I were playing square ball. As we passed the ball between us, I told them that I was moving. I had told them earlier that there was a chance that my mom would get married, but now it was official.

They didn't say very much during that recess. I filled the silence with idle chatter about how great everything was going to be when my mom got married. I was spitting out the same words that my mom had said to me so many times before. "Bob is a great person. We are going to live in a big house and Bob said I can get a dog." I chatted away as if to convince them (and myself) that I thought it was all going to work out. On the last day of school, I took a lot of pictures and we all promised that we would write.

CALM BEFORE THE STORM

That summer, we moved into an apartment as planned. It was a quiet summer. I liked our apartment, the carpet was a soft yellow-gold color which matched my bedroom furniture.

My mom was working hard at her mall productions. My sister and I spent most of our days swimming in the pool at our apartment, and our evenings were spent at Bob's house getting to know him and his children. We were all preparing for the wedding.

By this time, my sister and I had less and less in common. We were two years apart and we fought hard to create our own identities. We were involved in completely different activities, both at school and out of school; but the divorce, in its own way, helped to build a bridge between the two of us. Even with our differences, there were times every now and then when we would share something between us that seemed to make up for all the times that life got in the way of our love.

One morning, I woke up to the sun streaming through my window. I realized that I had overslept and jumped out of bed to see what was happening outside my bedroom door.

The apartment was completely silent. All signs of life were gone. As I looked in each room, I wondered where Shawn could be. It was too cold to go swimming, and I knew that she wouldn't have gone to work with my mother without telling me first.

Fifteen minutes had passed and I started to get worried. When half an hour had passed, I felt sure that something had gone wrong. I didn't know exactly where my mom was that morning so I didn't know where to call. We always had a list of numbers to call in case of an emergency; it was just a matter of finding the right one.

Finally, the door opened and my sister, her hands filled with bags, came through the door.

I said, "Shawn, where have you been?"

Seeing my worried expression she said, "Didn't you see my note?"

She picked a small piece of paper off the counter and handed it to me. The piece of paper said, "Shari, I went to get breakfast down the street, I'll be right back." All that worry for nothing!

These were great times. My sister, the oldest, would take money out of the change jar in our cupboard and walk all by herself to a nearby restaurant to get us breakfast. I liked it when she did this because it made me feel that she was taking care of me. I would never have had the courage to walk down the street to that restaurant alone. It was times like these that made me feel like she was the strong one; that I could lean on her and she could hold me up.

Shawn and I didn't talk about the pain of divorce. We seldom shared our feelings about anything deeper than the surface. I think both of us knew that if we did, the tears may never have stopped. So this was our way of communicating. She would bring me breakfast and I would clean her room sometimes or clean the house when she didn't want to. It might not have been perfect, but somehow we learned how to cope with the whirlwind of our lives and still manage to take care of each other, even if it was in the smallest of ways.

SCOTTY

That summer, Bob held true to his promise and found a dog for me that was unlike any other I had ever seen. He was a misfit just like me.

We found little Butterscotch in a box behind a barn at the fair near our cabin. They were giving the puppies away which was no big surprise. The poor little dogs were covered with fleas and were probably too young to be removed from their mother. Since they were going to be given away anyway I was glad that I could take one.

We decided to call him Butterscotch because that was his color - "Scotty" for short. He was no bigger than the palm of my hand and he had to drink from a baby bottle for a few weeks until he could handle solid food.

The owner of his mother said that he was a mixed bag of breeds. He was part cocker spaniel and poodle, plus some other things which we never figured out. My mom said that his mother was really ugly, with a big huge nose. My dog was very tiny and had little paws, so I never feared that he would grow to be big. I wanted a little dog that needed me to care for it.

I took care of Scotty, that flea-infested little fluff ball. I ended up with as many flea bites as he had. I washed him in flea soap and fed him with a bottle, and soon he became my constant companion.

Scotty was a great source of humor. As he grew so did his nose - and he had a big one. Then there were his teeth. His lower jaw stuck out about a fourth of an inch longer than his upper jaw. He looked like he was mad and growling all the time. In fact, he would have been scary if he wasn't so small. He had a big nose, a tiny head, an under bite, big burly shoulders, and a tiny back.

Animals have the most soothing effect when you are hurting or lonely. I could talk to my dog when no one would listen, and play with my dog when no one else was around. The great thing about animals is that they love you unconditionally. They don't talk back or care about your shortcomings. They just love you. That is what I needed then, something to love and someone to love me. I needed a purpose, and my dog needed me. It seems like such a simple thing, but when things were crazy at school or at home, I had a friend that would wait until I came home from school and run to me when I called.

I spent most of my sixth grade year with Scotty, running in the swampy, undeveloped area next to our house. It was just like the times that I had spent exploring the area near our townhouse the year before. The quiet times watching the horses in the pasture or just walking alone in silence were good for me. That is when I would sort everything out. Now, I had someone to walk with. Scotty was a nice distraction in a turbulent time.

STEPKIDS

That summer we became a stepfamily. That is so easy to say, but anyone who has ever formed a family with kids from different marriages knows that it is far from an easy task to make things run smoothly.

Mom tried very hard. She wanted peace to be in our lives - consistency, happiness, and love. My mom always tried to give that to my sister and me, and she would do no less for her new-found children.

I liked our family the way it was before. My mom, on the other hand, thought having two more children was wonderful. She came into that situation as she did with so many others, with excitement, ideas, and never doubting that everything was going to work.

Had she been tentative with these new children or demanded that they call her "mother" or push them to become attached immediately, they would have kept her at arm's length for a long time. Instead, she entered their lives like the Pied Piper whistling a happy tune. They were drawn to her because she allowed them to come to her when they were ready.

Yes, there were initial testings as each person checked the

situation out. In the end, the Pied Piper won. My stepbrother and stepsister grew to love my mom, if not as a mother, as a friend.

My mom came into a dreary house, a dark, sad house, where my stepfather and stepsister Jennifer had been living since his divorce, and she opened it up to life again. With our furniture and the few pieces they had, she turned it into a very nice, comfortable home. She opened the windows and let in the light, and she put flower arrangements in the dark corners of every room.

My mom made sure that a room was built for my sister and me before we moved in so that we could have our own place to live. The rooms were small; to get to my sister's room you had to walk through my room. I didn't care as long as we had our own space. Having your own space is very important when blending a family. Had we been forced to share everything with a sister and brother whom we had not had time to get to know, I think it could have caused some additional friction.

My mom not only transformed the main living areas of the house, she also transformed the bedrooms of my new brother and sister from downright ugly and gloomy to places where a kid would like to go. My mom worked particularly hard to transform Jennifer's room, for she would be living with us full time. She even started a doll collection for her. The collection lined a wall in her room and became Jennifer's favorite possession.

My stepbrother Timmy seemed to be a fairly well adjusted child. He went between our house and his mother's house with relative ease. He was a cute kid, happy it seemed, and he accepted the situation without many problems. I think his only problem was the fact that he now had three sisters bossing him around rather than one.

Jennifer, on the other hand, had many problems going on all at once when we came into her life. She was a beautiful girl but had a terrible self-esteem problem. She was overweight, unpopular and struggling with school because of undiagnosed learning problems. I think there were many problems in her life, some of which I can only speculate about, but the most destructive and painful was her rather volatile relationship with her mother. They loved each other in the only way that they knew how, but a connection was just not there. To top off an already difficult relationship with her mother, when Jennifer's parents were divorced, there was a harsh custody battle. Because of his age, Timmy was placed with his mother but Jennifer was given a choice. She chose her father and the gap between her and her mother widened.

I know Jennifer wanted her mother's love more than anything. Her mother was an attractive, slender person, and Jennifer wanted to be like her.

Maybe that's what drew me to her. I too searched for love, especially from my father. I could understand that desperation that drives you to please; and then when you fall short, there is a feeling of utter despair.

When we came into that household, my mom worked especially hard to smooth the pain that Jennifer felt. We all worked together to encourage her to lose weight and helped her to find clothes that would fit her at a price she could afford. These were changes that Jennifer wanted to make but was either afraid or didn't know how before we came into her life.

I became a little sister who looked up to Jennifer. I don't think many people had ever looked up to her before. Shawn became Jennifer's buddy, a friend, a person who could understand what Jennifer was going through. It was from Shawn that Jennifer would learn to raise her voice from no more than a whisper to a normal level. Jennifer watched Shawn and looked up to her. Shawn gave Jennifer courage in the same way that Shawn had made me feel strong and popular, just by being her sister and by being in her presence. She knew how to maneuver through life and both Jennifer and I watched, trying to figure it out.

Things got easier after the initial transition. Each of us took on our new role. My mom was everyone's mother, Bob was the new dad, Shawn was the older sister - not in age but in strength, Jennifer was the middle sister (although she was two years older than Shawn), and I was truly the younger sister. Now I wasn't just tagging behind Shawn, I was tagging behind Shawn and Jennifer. I gained a sister, brother, and father, but it was Jennifer and Shawn who got close. I was several years older than my stepbrother and didn't know my stepfather at all. So, even with all these new people in my life, I still felt alone.

There was still something missing in our new family. It was as if we were playacting, like it wasn't real. The role which seemed most unrealistic was Bob's. There was a time when I can say that I needed him. Maybe not as a father, but as a person in my life. But he was hard to get close to. I felt unsure when he was around because I couldn't tell how he was feeling.

Rather than letting his emotions show like my mom did, he tended to keep things inside. There would be tension filling the house for awhile. We knew something was wrong, but we just didn't know what. Then in sporadic outbursts, he would let everything go. Following the anger, we would all be left wondering where it all came from and when it would happen again. My mom would then set to work trying to smooth things over.

He was a big man. The kind of man that can either swallow you up in his arms in a wonderful bear hug or make you feel small in his presence. I learned to respect him, but I did not love him.

I can't say that we were ever physically abused by my stepfather, but there were times when the tension in the house was so thick that you could have cut it with a knife. There was a set of rules that all of us must go by, except for him. His wrath was strong and unpredictable. I learned to approach cautiously and to trust Bob with great reservations.

The most important point of this whole transition phase is the part that is still confusing even to me. I was a very self-conscious child, totally unsure of my appearance and my ever changing adolescent body. I was on the verge of puberty. I was a shy, extremely private child from early on. I think if my father and I had a touching kind of relationship, I would have found it more comfortable to be around a man and not feel strange. Instead, I learned to feel protective of myself and afraid that if someone got near me in some way, it was wrong, or that if given the chance, that person might hurt me. I didn't feel this with my father, but I felt wary of every other male person that was close to his age.

Because I was still young, I was around the house every day after school and in the evenings. My mom wanted me to like Bob so much that she would encourage me to drive with Bob to the grocery store, or to any number of places when an errand needed to be done. I wanted to say, "No, I don't want to go," but I didn't want to disappoint her. She thought that by doing this, we would bond and become close. Instead, I found myself feeling afraid. I didn't know Bob, I didn't feel comfortable with Bob, and I honestly didn't like being alone with Bob in any way, shape or form. Nothing ever happened, but I continued to be afraid and unsure in Bob's presence.

My mom now realizes that she made a mistake by pushing me to like the person she loved. Everyone needs to understand that a child like me with so many problems, someone who is searching to be loved, who can be easily manipulated and told that they aren't good enough or that everything is their fault, is the perfect target for abuse. Let time build the relationship rather than forcing it. Listen to your children and especially to a timid child. Be open so that they can come to you.

My fear of men, whether a teacher or a family friend, was a result of not having a stable relationship with my father. It kept me from trusting anyone who would possibly be a father figure in my life. Trusting meant the possibility of rejection, that I might lose them or disappoint them as I felt I had done with my father. It also meant that they could hurt me in ways that I could never say.

CHAPTER
9

SIXTH GRADE

During my fifth grade year, I had gone to a rural school set back in a little town outside of Seattle. Where you bought your clothes was last on the list of priorities among me and my friends. The school that I went to in sixth grade and the whole district that we lived in was quite different. The kids there had a lot of money. Their houses were some of the biggest I had ever seen in my life. In general, if any of them wanted something, they could buy it. So it is no wonder that I didn't exactly fit right in. We wouldn't have been considered poor in most neighborhoods, but we were in this one.

It didn't take me long to understand how ostracized you could feel wearing K-mart tennis shoes in a rich neighborhood. The kids in my class and those who surrounded me at school had the priciest duds on the rack. The mention of a "Blue Light Special" sent shivers down the spine of these youngsters of the "Rich and Famous." Vain or not, my family couldn't afford Nike's, so I just settled for ripping the Traxx labels off my shoes, hoping that nobody would know the difference. But these kids were not only rich, they were very astute at telling the difference between leather and vinyl. I came to school in my unlabeled shoes and they said, "Those are K-mart tennis shoes, you just ripped the Traxx label off of them. Right?"

In sixth grade I was still a ninety-eight pound duckling. I was so thin that I had to buy all my clothes from the children's department, which fit me though the pants were always a little short. At this point, my face was breaking out with lightening speed and no drugstore remedy seemed to work. I had ponytails that were so tight they made my eyes squint. And on top of it all, I wore K-mart tennis shoes. I was your classic nerd. Five foot, six inches tall with high-water pants, zits, Coke-bottle glasses, and K-mart tennis shoes. Now isn't that an incredible mental picture.

When you look in the mirror and are frightened by your own image, you walk around thinking that everyone else will be frightened, too. You are confident in only one thing, that everyone must think as little of you as you do of yourself. Because you think this, you actually read laughter and criticism into each person's expression, and meanness into each person's words. Everywhere you go, you hate yourself, so you are sure that everyone else does, too. Everything bad that happens to you isn't a fluke, it is your destiny. You expect bad things to happen and even sabotage yourself just to prove that the world hates you as much as you hate yourself. Isn't it amazing what a few zits and K-mart tennis shoes will do to your self-esteem! It would be great if it were that simple. The truth is, my sadness and my destructive image of myself had taken years to develop.

Since I had this thought process about myself and the world, it is logical that I would be devastated when I was not put into what was called, "the sixth grade wing," where all the other sixth graders in my school were. Instead I was placed into a split fifth/sixth grade class in a completely different wing from the other children my age. I think there were maybe five to six other sixth graders in my class and the rest were fifth graders. The remainder of the wing contained second and third grade classrooms. For the whole year, the sixth graders in my wing were excluded from participating in the same activities with the other sixth graders in the school. When this happened, it confirmed everything for me. I was dumb, so I was separated. I was ugly, so I was removed from the beautiful people. I was unpopular, so I couldn't be near those who where popular. It was the resource room syndrome of separation all over again. I was bad, so I was taken away from the good.

Let me just preface my next statements with this comment, "It was a going to be a rough sixth grade year." My home life was a mess, I missed my Dad, I had a major blemish problem, I thought everyone was laughing at me, I thought I was the ugliest person in the world, should I go on? Well you may be asking yourself, could it get much worse? Unfortunately it did get worse. I survived it, but it was a bumpy ride.

To save time, I'll just cut to the chase. With all the other things going wrong in my life, someone saw fit to assign me to a teacher who, the previous year, had been fired from the school that I was attending. He was going to sue the school, so they let him come back to teach. Now, doesn't that instill confidence in his classroom manner and teaching abilities? I heard the story rumored at the beginning of the year and I wondered why they were going to fire him. Once my sixth grade year started, I began to suspect that the reason may have been the amount of time he spent teaching sex education. No question about it, sex education was very interesting. In fact, the only information I retained from the whole year was the ongoing, in-depth, sex education material our class was taught. Not to make light of the situation, but I really could have used more education in spelling and math.

I had so many other problems going on in my life, I was the classic at-risk kid who needed help! Instead, I spent the whole year learning where babies come from.

When we did turn to a subject that was academic, I found myself floundering each and every day. My classroom that year was considered an "open concept classroom" where each student was supposed to go at his/her own pace. I went at my own pace and didn't learn a thing. Do to this open concept and the fact that my teacher was almost completely unresponsiveness to the needs of the students in his class, I constantly was left asking the part-time teacher's aide how to do my work. You see, when my teacher wasn't teaching sex education, he was preoccupied and distant. He spent most of his time in a corner of the room drinking tea. The open concept classroom allowed him a lot of free time to do this. This scenario depicting my teacher in one corner and me struggling in another is the way I remember my sixth grade year. I needed intense teaching, a resource room, and someone to help me. Instead, I felt completely ignored and denied the kind of help that I needed to progress. My teacher didn't want to be there, the open concept idea was just a mask for a free for all, and I was lost somewhere in the middle of it.

In this open concept classroom, the room became disorganized and disruptive. With everyone going at their own pace, some people would finish their work before others and would be allowed to play games or do other activities. This left those who were the slow learners, like me, struggling to learn amid the sound and movement of a busy room.

The idea behind the open concept led people to believe that it encourages the child to work on his own. Instead of the teacher teaching a lesson to the whole class, each of us were to go at our own pace in our textbooks. Again, for those who were quick learners and self-starters this was fine. But for those of us who had learning problems of any kind, it left us with books and no instructors.

Because of my challenges, I needed a teacher to teach me with oral instructions and examples rather than just written ones, constant eye contact, information given in repetition and in small increments, and quiet - none of which was available in my classroom.

I learned to hate almost everything about school that year. I was losing all hope that school was a place where I could succeed. I was squeaking by in class, but nobody seemed to notice. Because nobody else cared, I stopped caring. The year before, my schoolwork was highest on my list of priorities. By sixth grade, I found myself becoming despondent about school. I felt so tired in the morning that my feet would drag as I made my way to the bus stop to face another day.

I don't remember worrying that I would flunk out anymore. Certainly not out of this classroom anyway. It seemed impossible to flunk out. Even our grading system was designed to lower stress and allow people to go at their own pace. It did. I don't remember getting graded on anything the whole year. The fear that someone would come along and take me out of the school or hold me back had long since come and gone. I was more under the impression that nobody really noticed me.

I learned to look like I was doing my work, live for recess, and pray for the bell to ring. I sat in the back of the room, hid behind my book, and acted like I was reading. By the end of the year, I was still asking the same questions I had at the beginning. The teacher's aide thought I was just a slow learner; the teacher didn't notice.

HOLDING ON

Dealing with this terrible classroom set up and coping with my troubled home life sent my already low self-esteem plummeting! On the outside, I played the good little girl - going to school, staying quiet at home, talking the talk of a child my age - but I was at one of the two lowest points of my life.

Just as an anorexic gets a delusional image of herself in the mirror, I had a highly critical and distorted picture of myself. The years of being called "four-eyes" and "stupid" had finally gotten to me. I hated everything about myself. I thought I was the ugliest, dumbest person in the world.

My way of dealing with this image of myself was to avoid me at all costs. How do you avoid yourself you ask? Easy. First, you learn to avoid cameras. Why reproduce such an ugly image. I didn't want my picture taken. In fact, I only have one picture of myself from that whole year. I had school pictures taken twice and hated both sets, so I threw them away. If you wanted a picture of me, you had to take it quick and then hide it or it would be in the garbage.

Second, when you get up in the morning, you don't turn on the lights. I had a window that ran along the top part of one of the walls in my room, and on a good day there was enough light to get dressed by. If there wasn't, I just felt my way around the room.

I would lay out my clothes and my book bag the night before so that I could find things easily in the dim light. If I didn't have time to lay out my clothes before going to bed, I could still get dressed in the dark because I had everything hanging in my closet in color order so that I could just pick things out and they would match.

Third, I avoided all mirrors. I learned how to brush my teeth, wash my face, and apply mascara and makeup without the aid of a mirror. I would open up the medicine cabinet when I came into the bathroom and close it when I left so I wouldn't have to see myself. I developed a routine that made it possible to avoid all the mirrors in the house, and if I did need to look at my image, I would stand far enough away from it, or take off my glasses, or dim the lights so I couldn't see my blemished skin.

Other people might have looked at me and said, "Oh Shari,

you aren't ugly!" "Thanks Grandma, but why don't I have any friends? Why don't guys look at me?" I became more and more self-conscious and I was convinced that everyone was laughing at me. You can hate yourself that much.

When you feel this way, there is a tendency to hold onto one dream, one thing that you think will change everything if you could just make it happen. All my life I had wanted to be smart. I now felt that dream was completely out of reach. I couldn't change my brain, but I still had a hope that I might be able to change the outside of me. My most heartfelt goal was to be able to look into the mirror one day and see my face without glasses. I thought those glasses were the main reason why people looked at me and thought I was different. It was the last outward sign of being the first grade reject that I had once been and still seemed to be. I would look at my glasses and think, "When I get rid of these, people will accept me."

CONTACT LENSES

I was scheduled to see a new optometrist, he was supposed to be the best. I waited for that appointment with more anticipation than anything that year. Everyone else had said no, but I was sure this doctor was going to give me contacts. He was supposed to be able to fit even the most difficult patients' eyes with contacts. I believed so strongly that he could help me achieve this goal, I told the kids at school that soon I was going to get contact lenses.

When the long awaited appointment finally came, the doctor began to examine my eyes. When the exam was over, my mom stood next to my chair - she knew how important this was to me. Sadly, we listened as the doctor began to tell us that I would never be able to get contact lenses. I started to cry. That doctor was my last hope. I could hardly get control of myself. My mom watched as I sunk low in the chair. I thought then that I would be wearing glasses for the rest of my life.

My mom and I walked into the frames room. Once again, here I was, picking out another set of ugly frames to hold my thick lenses. I couldn't be consoled. My mom held up all different kinds of frames to my face, trying to cheer me up. But each one looked like the other, clunky and unattractive. She picked out a large pair of blue plastic frames and suggested that I tint the lenses a nice, deep blue. I passively agreed. For the rest of the year, I looked like a spaceman or a throw back from the sixties. You know those times when your mom says, "Oh, but they look so good!" and you want to say, "Mom, please, I'm in enough pain as it is. Not only do I look like a jerk, but I look like a jerk with big, blue-tinted glasses!"

I hated those glasses more than any pair I ever had. My image of those glasses was as exaggerated as my image of myself. That summer, I would try again to get contacts. Until then, I had sleepless nights dreaming that I would be wearing those embarrassing blue glasses to the bus stop for the rest of my life.

ONE FRIEND

Cammie sat leaning back in her chair the first day I walked into class. She was half my size with hair that went all the way down her back. She was tougher than I was. She would talk back and sass people in a way that I actually admired. She was strong, with a snappy personality, while I sat in silence and watched the world go by.

She looked me up and down that day - from my ponytails to my cheap tennis shoes. I didn't think she liked me and certainly thought she would never be my friend. There were so many reasons why we shouldn't become friends, and yet somehow we did.

It was a strange relationship because we were so different. Yet, I think we were drawn to each other because of our differences. She was so sharp and smart. She walked through life knowing she was great, while I tended to walk around feeling weak and unattractive. Being around her exhilarated me. Life didn't scare her. She made me laugh and I looked forward to seeing her everyday. Cammie became my only reason for going to school.

I had been so afraid that I wouldn't have any friends, but the girl with all the right clothes and the right hair liked me!

We hung around together every day at school, gossiped on the phone after school, and went places together on the weekends. Being with her made me feel daring and happy. She was loud and outspoken, and riding on her coattails gave me strength.

The most memorable thing that Cammie and I ever did together started out as a scheme to get out of going outside for recess. We used to come up with every excuse imaginable to get the teacher's permission to stay in at recess when it rained. The teacher often let us, but pretty soon we went over our limit. We needed an incredible idea to save us.

I think it was me who decided that we should put on a show, and it was Cammie who did the fast talking. We convinced our teacher that we were working on the "Shari and Cammie Joke Show" and that if he let us stay in during recess to practice, we would perform for the younger children at our school. He agreed, and we set out to work.

The room next to ours became our workshop. The desks and chairs that lined the walls of the room became our props. We found a divider to become our back drop; a platform in one corner would become our stage. The once hair-brained scheme that had been thought up to save us from the playground and the rain, had become a project that neither one of us could wait to start working on during recess.

It was appropriately named "The Shari and Cammie Joke Show" because that's what we did - we told jokes. Cammie had a few, I had a few, and together we had enough for about a fifteen-minute program. My mom had some clown suits that we wore for costumes. The props in the room weren't fancy, but nothing a little butcher paper and sparkles couldn't fix.

Before we performed for everyone, we realized that with only two people in the show, it would be difficult to make our entrance a surprise. This was a dilemma, but not for long!

Among the other strange events of my sixth grade year, I had decided to take the snare drum as my instrument in school. Of course, I could have played piano or the flute, but instead I chose the snare drum, which meant lugging that stupid twenty-pound case to the bus stop twice a week. I decided to give up the drums by the end of the year when I found that reading music for the drum was no easier than reading it for the violin. I was also sick of carrying the case.

The only good thing from my short snare drum career was that I was able to play a long drum roll. So, with the help of a tape recorder, Cammie and I were able to introduce ourselves in quite the Vaudeville fashion. The drum roll sounded and got louder and louder as we yelled in unison, "The Shari and Cammie Joke Show - Yeah, Yeah!" This musical introduction was the height of my drumming career.

Our show even had choreography. Both of us had seen the movie, Charley and the Chocolate Factory, and we had memorized the words to the "Oompa Loompa Song." We started our show by bobbing up and down behind our backdrop, singing the "Oompa Loompa Song" and telling jokes. Cammie and I sang "oompa loompa doopity, we have another riddle (sometimes we would say joke) for you." I would say the first part, she would say the second. Whoever was left standing when the song was done popped down behind the backdrop, and the other person jumped up and gave the punch line. After every joke, we would both pop up and say, "Yeah!" and make noises with our kazoos. Even if the crowd didn't like our act, we made so much noise that we couldn't tell.

The show went on with jokes and skits. For the finale, we sang the theme song from the Lawrence Welk Show. For those of you who can't remember that song it went something like this: good night, sleep tight, and pleasant dreams to you, here's a wish, and a prayer, that every dream comes true, and now till we meet again, adios, au revoir, auf wiedersehen, goodnight!

Cammie and I put our arms around each other and swayed as we sang our last song. It was a hokey song, but the words fit. After the song, we threw confetti and bags and bags of balloons all over the audience.

Several classes of younger kids signed up to see the show. Some teachers turned us down thinking we were crazy for asking them to take time out of their busy day to come see a joke show, but others accepted and we gave them a choice of show times.

Our class was the first to see it and everyone liked it. Then came all the other classes. Some of the kids liked our jokes, but most kids liked the balloons, the confetti, and the excuse to be out of class.

When the show was all over, Cammie and I were both sad. It had given us something to think about and plan for. Once it was over, we were back to recess like everyone else. We cleaned up the spare room, vacuumed up all the confetti and returned the furniture to its original positions. It was over, but I didn't forget that joke show experience for a long time. I learned more from it than anything else that year.

I had a friend in Cammie. We had planned something together, worked hard on it, and it had turned out well. But just when things began to look up for me, my teacher did something which plunged me into the saddest time of my sixth grade year. I have to believe that his actions were not done out of malice. I have to believe that he, like all of my teachers, did the best they could with what they knew. But when I was twelve years old, with a self-image that was so low, and a view of the world that was already bleak, what he did seemed cruel to me.

Even though there were many things I did not like about my teacher, he was my teacher and I gave him my respect and attention. Remember, I was the good little girl, never stepping out of bounds, always wanting to please. Sadly enough, I feel that my teacher knew this and that I longed for his praise and approval. He knew that I had few friends, with my only close friend being Cammie. Without her, I would be isolated.

One day, my teacher sat in his usual chair, drinking tea. He never seemed to have any paperwork or other things to do. He sat during our reading time and observed the class over his steaming mug. For no apparent reason, and without any warning, he called me up to his desk.

I sat and listened as he told me in a monotone voice (with a smile on his face) that it wasn't healthy to have just one friend. He felt that a person should have many friends. He said, "I know you and Cammie are close, but I think you should have other friends. Spend time with other people, Shari."

140

The words were blurred. I couldn't believe what I was hearing. He had no right to tell me who I could be friends with or how many friends is right for a girl my age. I was angry inside, but on the outside I was frightened, afraid to speak out. Was he serious? Was he going to tell Cammie that we couldn't be friends anymore? Would she listen? What am I going to do?

I begged him through my tears to please not tell Cammie. I needed her, she was my best friend. I said, "Cammie will have other friends, she does have other friends. Who will I have?" I kept repeating myself, and he just smiled and told me to pull myself together and to get some tissues from the bathroom.

I cried and cried in the bathroom. "Pull myself together," he said. Right! I'm in the middle of the worst year of my life and the only thing holding it together is the fact that I have one friend. And now, that was being taken away from me.

When I finally returned to the room, Cammie was sitting where I had been just moments before. She barely glanced at me when I entered the room. She looked shocked, but she didn't cry. I'll never know what my teacher said to her, and not knowing was worse than knowing. I imagined that he was telling her that she shouldn't hang around with a dumb, ugly girl like me, that she could have anybody for a friend. At that point, my mind was thinking only of the worst.

Cammie and I were not friends after that day. We didn't speak of what had happened and we avoided eye contact. Cammie went on just like I knew she would, she had other friends. I was alone.

I cannot trivialize this event in my life. I don't remember ever feeling so alone. I couldn't imagine who gave him the right to tell me who could and couldn't be my friend, to meddle in my life? For me it wasn't a matter of expanding my horizons and finding new friends. No one else would be my friend. Don't you see, couldn't my teachers see, I didn't have anyone else! A stronger child could take a blow like this. After this episode, I can honestly say that I didn't want to get up in the morning anymore, I didn't want to live. Whatever his intent, I will never believe that what my teacher did was justified, and I will never forget the pain and the length of time that it took me to recover from it.

When I felt alone and needed help, I had no one to go to at that school. I felt isolated in the farthest wing from the office. I didn't know any other teachers, nor did I know if there was a counselor who could help me. I didn't even know where the nurse's office was. No one ever came to our room and observed. I never even knew if there was a vice-principal, and until I inadvertently broke a rule one day on the playground, I had never seen the principal.

I didn't just block out the names or the faces because it was a painful year; I don't remember their names or faces because I never met any of these people or knew if they existed. My pain went inside where it festered and grew. On the outside, I didn't bother anybody; on the inside, I was dying. Sometimes I would think to myself, "Why doesn't anyone come and help me? Have they read my file? Do they know I'm here?" Apparently no one did know me. I was one of the masses of faces that passed through the hall and by the office doors, lost in the crowd. I was desperate for some help, but no one saw me.

We get angry at the students who act up in class and yell, scream, or kick over furniture. But they do get attention. We hear them. We yell at them, but at least we see them. Very often a principal, vice-principal, teacher, or counselor will see a student like that and know they need help. But what about the students who listen when told, are quiet, sit still, and don't break the rules? They look like they are normal from a distance, but if you dare to get close you will see their pain. My eyes in sixth grade reflected pain.

Many teachers and administrators either close the doors to their offices and weep or become hardened from the pain. They look at the numbers and the needs and feel that they can never be enough. But just one person can make a difference.

SOMEONE FOR EVERYONE

When I was little, because of my mom's work, we spent a lot of time at shopping malls. People-watching became my favorite pastime. Sitting on a bench and watching the people go by could keep me amused for hours.

Every now and then my mom would sit with me to rest, and we would watch the shoppers go by. We would see a lot of crazy-looking people, but the best was when we saw a couple who were wearing funny outfits or had outrageous hairdos. It was at those times that my mom would say, "There is someone for everyone."

In my gangly, pubescent years, I stood alone in the crowd. A wallflower of great proportions. At least compared to my sister, this was true. My sister was always being asked out and going steady with people, while I could only hope that someday the phone would ring for me.

But as my mom so often said, "There is someone for everyone." My someone was named Buddy. He was as odd as I was, maybe more odd, if that was possible. He too wore glasses and out-of-date clothes. His hair hung down in his eyes in a bowl cut, he carried an over-stuffed backpack and wore a hunting vest. He wasn't a prince charming and I wasn't a princess. It was a match. I met him, ironically enough, through my sixth-grade teacher. Buddy had been in my teacher's class a couple of years before and for some unknown reason, Buddy considered him a friend. I learned later that Buddy may have come to our classroom the first time to see my teacher, but after that he came to see me.

The teacher didn't mind Buddy's visits. He was just another kid wandering aimlessly through the room. He wasn't interrupting anything because none of us were doing anything. Soon Buddy became a permanent fixture in our class.

It was just an "across the room glance" at first. Glasses to glasses. Pretty soon Buddy was talking aloud to the teacher in hopes that one of his stories would travel across the room and awaken me to his presence. Most of the time I pretended not to hear. Everyone in the class would make jokes about him, so I didn't want people to see that I might like him. Even though I knew he wanted my attention, I pretended not to notice him.

In time Buddy became a little bolder. He began walking nearer to my desk as I worked. I pretended not to notice but when there is a 185-pound eighth grader practically sitting on your desk, it is pretty hard not to notice him.

Finally, I gave in. I liked him and he liked me. I didn't really announce it to anyone, but it was obvious Buddy and I were an item. I thought we could just continue as we were. I could be quiet about it, and we could just see each other when he came to our classroom. It would have worked out that way if it hadn't been for all the teasing that I received both at home and at school.

Buddy was a definite outcast at the junior high. My stepsister and sister knew of him and told me to stay clear of him. They would give me the worst time at the dinner table, asking if I had been visited by Buddy that day. On one hand they were joking, and on the other hand I think they were genuinely worried that I might actually like him.

On my birthday, Buddy gave me a gold necklace with an etched Aquarius symbol. And on Valentine's Day Buddy, drenched by the pouring rain, came to our door holding a wet paper bag clenched in his fist. Apparently he had come a long way on his bike to give me a present. I was too embarrassed to go to the door. I also was afraid my sisters would find out and I would never live it down. I sent my mom to the door as I stood and listened.

"Ma'am, will you give this to Shari for me?" My mom took the wet bag and assured Buddy that she would. I felt badly inside as I looked out the window and saw him get back on his bike and ride down our driveway in the cold rain.

I should have gone to the door, I thought later. I shouldn't let what other people think keep me from liking Buddy. But deep inside, I knew that I cared what people thought. I hadn't ever had a boy look at me before, certainly not one who gave me a necklace or a bag of soggy candy. I had never had someone drive his bike through the pouring rain to see me either. It was wonderful to be liked by a boy, but awful to fear people would make fun if you liked him back.

No matter how much I wanted to like Buddy, facing the peer pressure was more than I could take. I stopped talking to Buddy when he came to our class, and I tried to avoid him at all costs. Eventually, Buddy stopped coming to our classroom and he didn't come by our house anymore.

I saw him again when I was a junior in high school and a cheerleader. I had transformed from the ugly duckling to the head of the class. He was the same old Buddy, but a little more rough around the edges. He had a beard and his hair was long. He traveled the country in a caravan following a cult rock group.

Buddy changed when he got older, and so did I. But my memory of us will always be the same. He was the first boy to notice me despite my differences. I can still picture him with the rain running off his hood and with a soggy bag full of valentine candy for me.

I guess Buddy may have started a trend. I thought no one in the world would ever like me, but soon another boy in my class, Ted, began to like me. Ted wasn't an outsider. He was a sixth grader just like myself and even taller than me, which is nice when you are the tallest girl in the class.

Ted made his feelings for me official when he presented me with a tin ring. I could have fit two of my fingers in it; but it was all very exciting, so I wrapped it with tape and wore it with pride.

One day a group of girls from the sixth grade wing came up to me at recess. I didn't know them but they seemed to know me and had a message from one of their classmates. These were the popular girls of the sixth grade wing, no less. Apparently a boy from their "in" crowd named Ron liked me.

It was near the end of the year and I was feeling bold, so I decided to break it off with Ted and take my chances with the popular crowd. (Relationship decisions in sixth grade are so deep!) That same day Ron asked me to go steady. I knew it wouldn't last, but that didn't seem to bother me. He liked me. There were only two days of school left and I was going to bask in the glory of being one of the sixth grade wing girls.

Isn't it funny how things change? The girls from the sixth grade wing weren't even nice to me. But at the time, being liked by the "in" crowd for a three day period seemed better than being loved by the outcasts for a lifetime. I wanted to hold onto this moment forever. I brought my camera to school on the last day so that I could take pictures of all of my new found friends. The only picture that I have of that day explains the whole story. It is the three "in" girls, standing in the grass making faces at my camera lens. The reason why they appear to be making faces is because when I took the picture, they were saying, "Hurry up, Shari. We don't have time for this." That says it all. Those girls didn't care about me, and I didn't care enough about myself to realize it.

THE TRANSFORMATION

The summer finally came, and just in time. I had survived the worst year of my twelve-year-old life. I felt no sadness as I packed up my papers and pencils in a box and got on my bus to go home. Summer had come and with it came peace.

I cannot remember what my report card said that year. I can't remember what most of them said. I was learning to put the teacher's remarks and the grades behind me. As long as I passed, that was all I cared about. I no longer cared about the tests; I no longer saved the papers except for a precious few. I was only interested in survival.

One thing I did save from the school year was a collection of stories that I wrote through a journal writing project that lasted throughout the year. The stories were about a girl named Kristy and her horse.

The writing project was designed to develop our creative writing skills. You could write about anything that you wanted to in these journals, and you could change subjects at any time. I decided not to change my topic and instead made it into a book of stories about Kristy. Writing in my journal helped me to escape. Kristy was me, living the life that I wished I could lead. Each new story took me farther and farther away from my own existence.

While other people wrote short stories on different subjects, I had a book with chapters, page numbers and a plot. It was while writing in my journal that I decided to be a writer - a dream I never shared with anyone.

Although the project wasn't graded, my teacher had periodic conferences with each student about our writing skills. He offered little encouragement about my writing. By the time the year was over, I put down my journal and wrote little, if anything, until I was almost nineteen. His lack of encouragement, combined with years of failures in the classroom in regards to my writing, plus my own frustrations with trying to write my thoughts on the page, made me feel that I was a bad writer and that it was useless for me to try to express my thoughts with pen and paper.

I had listened to countless people who year after year said, "Your writing is unclear, I don't understand what you are trying to say, your grammar is atrocious," and believed that because I didn't have perfect English skills, my ideas on paper were worthless. For years, I looked at my typewriter with fear and picked up a pen with dread.

But there was a writer inside of me. Sometimes in the quiet of my room I would write short stories or poems. Sometimes I would share my writings, but only with my mother. I knew that I was safe with her. Most of the time, I would read them to her because I knew that I could read through my funny writing and my spelling errors as if they weren't there. She used to encourage me and say, "Shari what a wonderful writer you are. Don't worry about your spelling, that can be fixed. Just keep writing."

My mother planted the seed in my head that I could write and that my stories were good. Her confidence kept the dream of writing alive for me.

I kept those Kristy stories. No matter how little praise I received for them, no matter how many spelling errors were present on every page, I was proud of that work and decided to save the only thing that I had to show for a whole year of school. I tucked those stories away in a box and hoped, despite what other people said, that someday I might be a writer.

I meet so many kids and adults who think that they are not good at anything. This is never true. The truth is that they probably have failed before and are afraid to try again. Maybe they were told sometime in their life, once or many times, that they were no good or lacked talent. Being good at something is not always immediate; those of us with learning disabilities have to work even harder to develop our talents and learn new skills to find what we are best at. In the end, we will find that, despite the challenge and assessments of others, we have much to offer the world.

PICKING BERRIES

When my Mom and Bob were married, Bob set up a system of chores and allowances for all the kids. My sister and I had rarely received an allowance in the past. Chores were something we just did.

On the other hand, we began working for my mom's company from very early on. There was always a job to do and she would pay us for work well done. I learned to work for my money at an early age, to save, and to shop wisely. I used to be shocked when a kid my age would tell their parents to buy them a thirty dollar pair of jeans or a forty-five dollar pair of tennis shoes. I wouldn't have thought of doing that; my mom provided the essentials for us and we worked to buy extras.

The system in our new house included dusting and vacuuming, laundry, and dishes. Each girl took a job and it rotated from week to week. We received ten dollars a week to do our chores and with that we paid for our candy, movies, and school clothes. I soon found that if I saved my money each month, I could buy the top of the line tennis shoes or two pairs of pants from the teen clothing store where the popular girls shopped.

After a bad year in sixth grade, I was determined that with or without contact lenses, I was going to fit in at school during seventh grade. I thought that if I just had the right cloths it would make all the difference. I planned to save my allowance all summer and buy school clothes with it. By the end of the summer, I would have about $100 dollars if I saved every penny. I realized that for me to buy the clothes I wanted, I would have to add to my allowance money some other way.

Bob told all of the kids that if we desired, we could stay with my stepgrandparents and pick berries in their fields to make extra money. It seemed like a great idea at the time. If the picking was good, they said we could make double in two weeks what we would make the whole summer in allowance. My sister balked at the idea but my stepsister and I got sucked in hook, line, and sinker.

I have to admit I was going to stay with my stepgrandparents primarily because they had two ponies. The thought of riding ponies for two weeks sounded so irresistible that I agreed to pick berries in the fields.

To make a long story short, the trip was a disaster. My stepsister and I would get up at 4:30 in the morning so that we could catch our bus to the fields. The only thing that woke me up was the cold morning air on my face as we walked to the bus stop.

At the bus stop, we experienced culture shock. Jennifer and I were from a rather sheltered background. We, wearing our freshly washed pants and pastel shirts, found ourselves face to face with the hooligans of the local juvenile delinquency hall. The kids were smoking, drinking, swearing, and fighting from the time that we got to the bus stop to the time we got home.

The bus driver, Marian, was as tough talking and mean as the kids on the bus. She treated us all like animals and swore as fast and as mean as the "lovely" children in her care.

For eight hours a day we sat under the hot sun in the muddy berry field and picked berries. While all the experienced pickers were going from one row to the next filling up flat after flat, Jennifer and I sat trying to get just one row done between us. Some of these kids had come out every year since they were old enough to walk and they knew what they were doing. Nobody told us what to do, so we just sat there and tried to do our best.

I learned a lot that summer. I heard language like nothing I had ever heard before. I saw drugs being sold out in the fields.

I saw a whole different side to life, and I knew I never wanted any part of it.

At lunch time we ate still sitting in the dirt, with filthy berry-juice stained hands. Yes, we could have washed them, but only by fighting everyone for the use of the one water spigot. And then there was the bathroom, if you could call it that. There was one outhouse in the field where we were picking. I made the decision early on that if I could possibly stand it, I would wait until I got home to go to the bathroom. I made this decision after seeing two large boys, the oldest of the workers, play a practical joke on one of the other pickers. These kids were so big that they could literally rock the outhouse, and could even knock it over if they wanted to. I was afraid that if I ever went in that outhouse, the walls would start rocking and I would find myself in the middle of the field with no outhouse around me. That was a strong deterrent to keep me from drinking anything out in the field.

Berry picking went from being a great money making proposition to being an awful experience. We didn't make the money we were told we were going to make. At most, both Jennifer and I made about fifty dollars each for two weeks' work. The bonus that we received at the end for sticking with the job amounted to about four dollars. Both Jennifer and I were extremely unhappy from the beginning and wanted to quit after the first week.

We called and asked if we could come home. Bob basically said, "Either you stick with the job or you are quitters." I don't think my mom had much to say about the whole thing because she would have allowed us to come home in a minute.

Even Jennifer's grandparents wanted us to continue. They sided with Bob and felt that we should finish the job; I couldn't understand why. My sister had taken over our jobs at home, and by the time we returned she had made more money than Jennifer and I put together. Why should we stay and do this awful job when it isn't teaching us anything except new swear words?

Even the lure of riding the ponies had lost its glimmer. My stepgrandmother wouldn't let me ride until I had finished eating dinner. By that time, I was so tired and it was so late that there was little time left to ride. I was getting frustrated and missing home more and more as the days passed.

The only good thing about the whole trip was that Jennifer and I had a chance to get to know each other in a way that I considered to be special. Before, it had been Shawn and her, and I was too little to participate in their gossip. Now it was our turn. I was the only one there for her to talk to. Talk we did. All day long we would inch along the strips of strawberry plants and talk about all kinds of things: family, relationships, and our futures.

She told me stories about herself and about what she wanted to do in the future. She even told me about her boyfriends, or those that she would like to have one day. I felt privileged to be let into her life like that, to be trusted with her secrets. I loved her before, but now there was something different. Something that I would hold onto in the years to come.

I had always thought that if I were an older sister, I would do things differently. I would talk to my younger sister, tell her things, and give her advice. My sister did that sometimes, but most of the time I was in the way. So this was a real treat; talking to Jennifer was like being a real sister for the first time. We didn't seem to experience the age difference or seem to realize that we were stepsisters then. It was just two sisters talking and laughing and loving each other. When we went home, we returned to our respective roles and places. Jennifer was close to Shawn again and I was just the little sister. But for a while, we had been equals.

Sometimes people lash out at the person whom they are closest to because they know that person won't leave them. Jennifer did that with my mom sometimes. My mom loved her but Jennifer would often lash out at her after a painful visit with her mother or after disagreements with her father. She knew my mom would still love her in the end and would stick with her through thick and thin. I was also the target of Jennifer's anger, usually just because I happened to be there at the wrong time. She knew I wouldn't leave her, so I was easy to pounce on.

When we were on our berry picking trip, Jennifer was deeply upset by the reaction that we had received when we called home and asked to quit our job. She felt that we were completely abandoned, without support, and that nobody understood the situation. Being called "quitters" was very painful. With all the other things that Jennifer was experiencing in her life, this was just one more blow. Our request was just another opportunity to be met with a retort of, "If you just tried harder... If you were more determined... If you were more like me, you wouldn't quit."

It was after that phone call that I tried to reach out to Jennifer and comfort her. She pushed me away and yelled at me. She was hurt and took it out on me. Then she shut herself in her room. She didn't come out for a long time.

Feeling hurt, I went to the pasture and rode the ponies for a couple of hours. When I came back, Jennifer handed me a letter, gave me a hug and apologized. I have held onto that letter for years. It is the only handwritten piece of Jennifer I have left. I keep it because even though she had a hard time expressing herself, the letter showed her feelings as much as possible for her.

Dear Shari,

I'm sorry. It's easier for me to write it than to say. I know that I bug you a lot. I think we are both tired. I really am glad that we both went berry picking. The one thing that I want most right now, is some appreciation from my father. It really ticked me that he wasn't proud of us for even trying. We deserve a lot more credit than we got. I love you as the sister I never had. Thank you for all of the nice things that you have done for me during this trip. No matter how much that we may fight, I'm not afraid to say I love you.

Love Always,
Jennifer (thanks)

I thought I knew Jennifer. Picking berries with her helped me to get closer to her and her thoughts. And yet, I don't think any of us could know exactly what she was feeling. There were things going on that only she could know. She had made several suicide attempts at this point. Her reasons were wide and varied. I could only see part of her pain. Sometimes I think to myself, "If I had just spent more time with her, maybe I could have saved her from the pain that she was going through." But she never let me close enough to even know how bad it was. I just knew that she seemed to be sad more often than not and that she desperately wanted love and approval from her parents.

Her pain was similar to what I felt during my parents' divorce. But I had always felt that somehow, someway, things would always get better. By this time in my life I was so caught up in my own survival that I thought Jennifer was just like me, that she too would get through and not give up. In reality, her letter to me (as were many of the things that she wrote, said, and did) was a cry for help. She was saying very simply, "Love me."

THE NEW ME

On my arrival back from my berry-picking adventure, my mom and I went to see a new eye doctor. He was a genius - he could fit my hard-to-fit eyes with contacts!

My mom knew how much I wanted contacts. Even though we had been turned down six months earlier, we started to think that maybe that doctor had been wrong. Thankfully, my mom was an optimist, and I had learned to always keep trying. We had heard so many discouraging diagnoses, many of which had proved to be incorrect. So we decided to try again.

By the middle of summer, I had a pair of contacts. It took me a long time to get used to my lenses. I walked around with my eyes scrunched up and my brow furrowed because they hurt so much. When I started school in the fall, people thought I was either angry or concerned all the time. People greeted me by wrinkling up their forehead and saying, "Hi, Shari! Are you concerned about something?!" I got used to it, it even got to be funny.

A pair of contacts and a new acne medication did wonders for my self-esteem. They may have been small changes, insignificant to someone else, but they made me hopeful again.

Jennifer and Shawn took me out shopping before school started. We went to the most popular store for teen clothes. The store had all of the latest fashions and styles. I started the school year with new clothes and a pair of genuine Nike tennis shoes. My sister then informed me that I couldn't go to "her" school with ponytails. She took out the rubber bands and clips that I wore and convinced me to wear my hair down. What a difference it made! I looked like a new person.

My life was now taking on a whole new order. Once I took care of the outside, it was time to tackle my next goal. Sixth grade had left me feeling like I could never achieve success in school. But getting a pair of contact lenses, when I was told that I would never wear them, made me think that maybe never isn't forever. I began to think that maybe failing at school didn't always have to be.

As the beginning of the school year came closer, I decided I wasn't going to hide in class anymore, I wasn't going to just get by. I wanted something more from myself.

I realized that I had absolutely nothing to lose. I had tried and failed, which didn't feel good. I had also failed to try, and that didn't feel good, either. I knew that I had survived failures and could again. But I didn't want to be a failure, I wanted what everyone else had - success. But to achieve, I would have to change.

CHAPTER 10

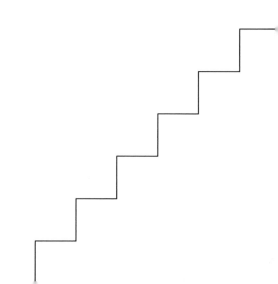

LEARNING A DIFFERENT WAY

This whole section is dedicated to helping students, adults, parents, and teachers to understand what alternative forms of learning are and how I began developing and using them. Most of my ideas that are shared here were developed in seventh grade and then refined over my years in school.

I hope each of you will find something helpful in this section; but most of all, I hope it expresses what I have always felt: that we all learn differently. No one way will work for us all. Take from my ideas and add your own. Soon you will have custom-made strategies for yourself and your study program.

From the first day of the seventh grade, I was filled with determination. I was determined to the point that I would cling to the desk and plant my feet on the ground. I made a vow to myself that this school year was going to be different.

Each year had taught me that trying to learn like the other kids in my class didn't work for me. I was different and I knew it. I just had to find a way to deal with my challenges and still be able to achieve. I decided to go back to the successful concepts that I had first learned in my third grade classroom and those concepts I had devised myself along the way to develop a custom-made study plan just for me.

BARRIERS FOR SAVING ENERGY

I came to class on those first days of school and managed to get a front row seat in almost all of the classes that had open seating. I knew that the first key to my learning was being able to see and hear what the teacher was saying and doing. Sitting in front took care of both of these things.

Even with my glasses, I found seeing things at any great distance difficult. I also found that sitting in the middle or back of a class left me unable to concentrate because there was movement and noise from the other students in front of me. When I sat up in front, I then had an unobstructed view of the teacher, the overhead projector, and the writing on the board; and I could hear all instructions and lectures clearly. My back literally became a wall to any noise or distractions behind me.

As a learning disabled person, I spent a lot of energy in just getting through a day. When I got home from school, I was totally exhausted and frustrated. Sitting up front allowed me to see and hear clearly, which in turn, allowed me to conserve some of my energy to put into other things.

When I tell learning disabled students to sit up front in class, they shake their heads and start to panic. They say, "I'm not going to sit up in front, someone might call on me." They have had a bad experience and want to hide in the back of the class and not be seen. They think if they hide long enough, people will forget they exist. True, they don't get called on, but they also don't learn as much and they don't get a participation grade. If you want a better grade, you need to let go of the fear of being called on and move yourself to the front of the room.

SURROUNDING YOURSELF WITH PEOPLE WHO WANT TO LEARN

There is another good reason for sitting up front. I found a different type of student sitting there - one who was more likely to be quiet and watch the teacher than those who sat in the back or in a corner. It seems that if you sit up front, it is because you want to learn. This is not always the case, but I found it to be true more often than not.

I figured out that although talking to the person sitting next to me was more fun than trying to learn, it wasn't going to help me pass the class. I had to remove myself from the people who would rather talk than learn; otherwise, I would have been easily distracted and pulled into the conversation. By moving myself to the front of the room, I was moving myself away from my old habits of hiding and talking to those around me, and putting myself in a place where I would have to pay attention.

Many of the kids that I meet have a group of friends who urge them on in class, encourage behavior that puts them in the hall and keeps them from learning and doing their work well. Learning disabled students must choose their friends wisely. They must move away from the back of the room and the friends that keep them from listening and understanding. I'm not blaming other people for my learning problems. I just know that to be successful in school, you have do what you have to do to achieve. If that means sitting up in front away from your friends, or coming to class when your friends say let's skip, do it!

By the time I reached seventh grade, I knew and had decided that my grades didn't belong to the person sitting next to me or even to the teacher. They were mine. I couldn't wait for someone to tell me what to do and which path to take, or to come to me with a silver platter and say, "Shari, here are the grades you always wanted." It doesn't happen that way. It is your choice and your determination that will give you the grades you know are possible to achieve.

HOW DO YOU KNOW WHAT STEPS TO TAKE?

Now that you are sitting up front and have removed yourself

from potential distractions, the next question is: how do I learn what is being taught? It is all a process of elimination, trial and error. What works best for you? Hearing, seeing, repetition, saying it out loud? Everyone knows generally what works best for them or could think of some things that they could do to help themselves to learn better, like sitting up in front, turning off the stereo while studying, using flashcards. Try things out and see what happens.

Some people won't try because they don't think anything will work. If, after you know that there are choices, you still feel that you don't want to try, then that is up to you. For me, the greatest handicap is being without choices. There is always a way - sometimes it just isn't obvious. You may have to search and try to ask questions of your teachers, or even of other students to see how they learn. There is a way for you to learn, you just have to find it.

Learning what worked for me was a slow process. I had to try many things before I found what study habits gave me the best results. In time, I found that repetition used in a multi-sensory way was the key to unlocking the doors to my brain. I had to see it, say it, write it, hear it, touch it, anything to understand the information. Once I learned the material, I had to figure out how to retain it. When I finally did retain the information, which took a lot of time, I then had to hope that my brain could hold up under the pressure of being called on in class or when taking a test. Sometimes I didn't do that well. Yes, it was embarrassing to make mistakes, especially in front of my classmates, but I had to let go of the failures and keep trying.

I had to learn how to raise my hand without fear of being called on. I was scared to speak out loud in class because I thought I might stumble through what I had to say, forget what I wanted to say, or repeat a question or make a comment that someone had already said. All of it was new to me. My fear of failure in the classroom didn't go away completely; but I found that every day I worked on learning strategies, it became easier.

Breaking out of your shell and trying new things is scary. But you have to do it. The longer you wait, the harder it is to get over that fear. Just try!

LEARNING HOW TO CONCENTRATE

I could sit up front in class, I could even build an imaginary wall around myself, but that still would not ensure that I could concentrate. In fact, concentration was one of the toughest processes for me to master. How do you tune out what you can't physically block out? At home, I had control and could turn off the TV and go to a room that was silent. At school, I couldn't do that.

I found that I had to develop a sense of concentration. I learned to plug my ears during a test by cupping my hands over my ears. I learned to sit in a cubicle at the library to keep myself from seeing distractions. I had to watch the teachers closely, read their lips, watch their motions, and say each word over again in my mind. At first I still found myself distracted, and I felt the need to look out the window and get away from my frustration. In time, my sense of concentration improved at home and in the classroom. But at first, it was sheer determination that kept me focused and concentrating, instead of giving into feeling disorganized and scattered.

To keep my concentration level steady, I learned that I could not do more than one thing at a time. My work space had to be free of clutter and distractions, especially noise. I learned that I could not do my studies during work time at school. I had to be in a room that was silent, which was usually not until I got home.

Because I had to take all my assignments home, I had to get plenty of examples and instruction ahead of time. I learned to get help with my questions before, during, and after school so that I wouldn't have to compete with the other kids waiting in line to see the teacher. Catching the teacher alone was a trick, but when I did, I learned so much more.

Concentration, to me, is more than tuning out the noise and distractions. I thought it was just that at first. In time, it became apparent to me that my ability to concentrate was determined by a lot of things, particularly the amount of sleep I had the night before, the time of day, how hungry I was, or if I had just eaten sugar.

When I was little, I would bounce off the walls all the time. As I got older, my hyperactivity was more controllable and easier to deal with. I was able to control my ability to concentrate and sit still in class when I did not eat sugar and processed foods, which made me feel jumpy, itchy and distracted. I also learned to eat three meals a day rather than snacking on junk food or eating candy.

Being hungry is just as bad as being full of the wrong kind of food. When I was hungry, I felt light-headed and out of touch. Some people can fast and skip meals and not feel disturbed, but I can't. What, when and how much I eat are all factors that I look for to help maintain my concentration.

Changing what you eat isn't a cure-all. Neither is changing when you eat. But if you find that eating certain types of foods makes you empty-headed, tired, or hyperactive, you may be allergic to or have a sensitivity to them. I take the time in the morning to eat a good breakfast. I eat nutritious food instead of candy at mealtimes, and I carry an apple or some almonds in my purse or pocket to maintain a steady energy level. See if it makes a difference for you.

I have also found that sleep makes a world of difference in how I am able to understand information. I know that I learn better in the morning, so I put my hardest classes first on my schedule. I am tired by the end of the day, so I put my easier classes in the afternoon.

I hear people say, "Well, I am a night person and you are a day person." Frankly, when you are in junior high and high school you don't have much choice about the hours you keep. Most schools start sometime around 8:00 a.m. If you stay up until midnight, you're right, you won't be a morning person at 8:00 in the morning. I love to stay up late. I do when I am not working or attending school. When I am in school, it is crucial for me to get eight hours sleep every night and even more before a test.

I find that my brain short circuits when I need it most if I pull an all-nighter for a test or stay up late before an early morning class. It seems like such a simple thing, but getting enough sleep will help you do better in school. Simple, but how many of us do it? You may be able to get a "C" on a test with four hours of sleep, but what could you get with eight hours? Do the work leading up to the test, then you won't have to stay up all night and go to school with a foggy brain. Get enough sleep all the time, and I'm sure you will see the difference.

HOMEWORK

Not doing my work at school meant that I came home with a lot of homework. I looked at that stack of books and it felt like I was facing a mountain. I felt frustrated before I ever began.

Again, knowing that no one was going to do my work for me, I had to find a way to deal with the frustration so that I could get my work done. I made a plan for myself to follow.

The first part of the plan was making sure that before I left school, I had a clear understanding of what was being asked me. Once you get home, you are on your own. Make sure that you have all the information that you need to do your assignments. Go ask the teacher for more examples so that when you get home, you won't get stuck. If you are embarrassed, it's alright to ask a question when no one else is around. I did. The main thing is, ask the question!

When I came home from school, I would do my chores or take a walk with my dog so that I could release some energy. Even though I was tired from the day at school, I still had a lot of nervous energy that kept me from being able to concentrate right away. I tried to drag out after-school projects for a long time, wanting to avoid hitting the books. But I knew that by late evening I would be falling asleep over my books, so I learned to start my homework about an hour after I got home from school.

Once I started my homework, the frustration began. Here are some things that I did which helped me to do my homework rather than avoid it: do something you like before you study and during your study breaks; make a schedule with rewards along the way; study for a certain amount of time, then give yourself a short break - this will help lower the frustration. The key is to stick with your schedule. You can't study for two minutes and break for five; you won't get anywhere. Start out with twenty to thirty minutes with a five minute break in between.

When I first started to learn how to study, I found it hard to sit for more than fifteen minutes without wanting to stomp on my books. Yes, everything in the world is more interesting in these initial stages than studying. If you want it, you will do it. In time, you will see that the longer you sit there, the easier it becomes. You will also find that as you learn to concentrate, to quiet the noise in your brain and to put your eyes into the book, you will begin to absorb more, faster. Everyone is different; you will need to make your own schedule, but it will get better.

Initially, your attention span might not be long enough to finish a project or an assignment between breaks; but over time, try to build yourself up to a point where you can finish one project before taking a break or moving on to another assignment. I found that finishing a project in one sitting, rather than dragging it out over a long period of time or switching from one thing to another, is a great way to keep your focus and reduce frustration while studying. You can't do that with a ten-page report, but with other assignments you can. I find it easier to finish what I start right away because each time I walk away from my books, I lose my place, my thoughts get scattered, and I feel disrupted. If I sit there and finish it, I can stay focused.

At first, sitting long enough to finish one project can be frustrating. You will find yourself wanting to move on to another project because that is how the learning disabled brain works; it is scattered and unorganized. But don't do it. Practice doing one assignment at a time and practice concentrating rather than drifting from one thing to the next while studying. You will see the difference.

When we get frustrated, we have a tendency to rush. Allow yourself the time to do good work. Nobody is really proud of a sloppy, half-completed assignment. I used to be embarrassed to hand in work like that. When my homework was sloppy, it was because I didn't allow the time to prepare and do it right.

If you're frustrated, take a break and come back to it. Allow yourself the time to finish, but finish it well. Give yourself time to read the directions. Read the directions at least three times - or until you fully understand them. I used to be in such a hurry to finish a test or an assignment that I missed important directions that would have helped me in the long run, so READ THE DIRECTIONS!

When you look at that stack of books, don't panic. Don't put it off either. The later it gets in the evening, the less chance that you have of finishing your work. Set a goal to be finished by a certain time - maybe the time that a certain TV show begins - so that you will have an incentive to get to work and get things done.

Start out with something easy that you know you can finish. I used to play games with myself. I would take a book out of the stack and start with the easiest assignment. I would finish it and then start building the "done" pile. I would then do the next easiest assignment just so that I could have at least two assignments on the "done" pile.

If I didn't do it this way and started out with the hard assignment first, I would get frustrated and never finish anything. The best way is to start easy and put the hardest assignment "in between." Don't save the hardest assignment until last. By then, it may be late and you will be too tired to start it let alone do it well. Put it in the middle so that you will still have energy left.

All of this is great, but what about a long project? It will take organization, orderly notebooks, and a clean, quiet work place. For long projects, you have to have a time schedule and a course of action that will lead you through weeks of work without cramming or rushing to get it done.

If you have to go to the library, it will take extra time. If you have to interview people for the report, it will take extra time. Allot a certain amount of time per day to a long project. I crammed to finish a report once and I ended up with a frazzled brain and a half-baked report. Take it step by step and leave a couple of days to prepare the final draft, to have someone proofread it for errors, and to type it.

I have heard some kids say, "Well, I can still get a D even if I cram." Fine, if that is all you want. Personally, I want more. I want what I know is possible. Don't settle for second best. Don't look at your friend finishing her work quickly and think that you can do that, too, and come out with the result you want.

I find the same thing is true when studying for a test. I have a short memory span, so it is better for me to study over a long period of time than it is to cram during lunch on the day of the test. I need more time to get the information into my brain, to retain it, and to remember it under pressure.

When you over-stuff a closet and then open the door, the contents fall out without any order or clarity. If you pack everything in and fold it, you will be able to open the closet door and take each item out when you want it, in the order you want it. That is what you have to remember when studying for a test. Do it step by step. If you do this, you will be able to remember the information better under pressure than if you had just studied the information an hour before. You will also be able to retain the information over longer periods of time and under pressure.

What if you are asked to retain the information for the final that will come at the end of the grading period? Do you think that cramming for a test will allow you to hold onto that information over a long period of time? No! You will be forced to relearn it again with the same stress that you went through before, with the same uncertainty and the same results or lack of them that you experienced when you crammed for tests.

Also, to help you prepare for a final exam, keep all of your old notes in a separate notebook divided by class. Don't throw anything away because you never know if you will need it again. To study for a final, set aside fifteen minutes a day to go over your notes or a section of your notes. Keep doing this until the final and you will find that when you reach the test date, you will have already done all the work. No pressure, no cramming, and a much better chance of a good grade.

Over the years, I have learned that many classes are cumulative, meaning that what you learn in the beginning sets the stage for what you will learn later on. You must understand the first steps of a concept to understand the full concept. You must keep up in your classes to get a passing grade. You can't do that by cramming. Learn the first part of the lesson rather than waiting until test time. I guarantee that you will be less frustrated and more likely to finish your assignments and pass the class if you take some initial steps at the beginning of the class. Study over a period of time, get help right away if you have problems, and keep all of your notes. Most important of all, set up a pattern and organize your homework and your routine for school.

ORGANIZATION

With learning disabilities, our brains are sort of scattered and muddled. Many of us are known as the absent-minded professor types, the ones who are always late and arrive without the proper materials for the class or without homework. Organization is our key to success.

Do you start a project in the middle or find it hard to decide what assignment to work on first? Are you often in trouble for not having your assignments in on time? Do you often go to class without the proper materials? Start by being organized. Make a list of all of the books and materials that you need to bring home from school. Have pencils, paper, and other supplies in your locker, your book bag and at home. If you don't have the materials, you can't get the project done. Also, make a list or keep a book of homework assignments, due dates, and test dates. This will insure that you will never be caught off guard for a test or project.

Next, when you sit down at the table, is everything in disarray? Are the papers coming out from all sides of your notebook from every direction? Are class materials filed in a divided way or is everything just meshed together?

When the area that surrounds you is messy, you will feel messy and out of control. When you make things more organized and patterned, your brain will calm down and you will be able to concentrate better.

Make your work area clean and neat, with no distractions to catch your eye. Organize your notebook by labelling each section. Get a hole punch and reinforcers so that nothing breaks out of your notebook and gets lost. Cover and label all your books. Use a different color of paper for each book so you don't grab the wrong one by accident.

Being organized does take more time. It also means that your grades will go up and that your teacher will no longer call you "the kid who is never prepared." The reward for your time is a better grade.

TEST ANXIETY

Almost everyone will experience test anxiety at least once in their lifetime. Everyone experiences it, but for those with learning problems, it can be an even greater source of stress. Test anxiety is fear. Fear of the unknown and what will be on the test; fear of not being able to remember what you studied. For a learning disabled person, add fear of filling in the blanks, spelling, and a whole host of other skills that plague us on a day to day basis but are magnified in a test situation. No one can take away your anxiety, but there are things that you can do to make taking a test easier.

Studying for the test is as important as what you do once the test is in front of you. I want to mention a couple of studying tips that are particularly useful. For tests that are based on a lot of reading material, the best thing to do is to read through the assigned chapters. The second time through the material, begin highlighting with colored highlighters the points that you think are important. The third time and each time following, read and do something else that involves your motor skills such as writing, or use vocal skills such as reading out loud to keep your mind focused on what you are reading. If you get too familiar with the information, you may zone out and not actually understand the words that are buzzing across the page; that is why you must combine another part of your senses while reading to keep yourself involved.

I usually begin by first reading through a chapter once. On the second reading, I highlight main ideas while listening to the chapter on tape. By the third or fourth time, I make a set of flashcards on that chapter that outlines and defines specific words and concepts that are important to that chapter. Once I have the flashcards, I go through the side of the flash cards which has the words or concepts and I define them both out loud and by writing the information down on a scratch piece of paper. This helps me practice recall of the information. Then I go through the other side of the cards, read the definitions to myself, and then identify the concept or word that definition refers to. During this step of the process, it is important to make sure that when you identify the word or concept, you also know how to spell it correctly. Say the words and the concepts out loud and write them down to practice spelling and recall. If you just read the book, it is very unlikely that you will truly remember what you have read. If you combine other senses such as hearing, speaking and writing, the information will be easier to remember, and studying will be more interesting.

One important thing to remember is that you should make flashcards and keep the information in the order that the book is in. As you learn the information on these flashcards, make a mental association of words and pictures as they are seen in the book. As you read your flashcards, think about what page that word was mentioned on, not the page number, but in the context in which it was mentioned and what picture was associated with it. Flashcards contain a small bit of information that serves as an outline. When you have learned the information from the book, then use your flashcards as your outline of the book and quiz yourself from them. After doing this, it will be easier to come up with answers on the test that relate to the book, even if it is a word or concept that you aren't familiar with. You will see a word and be able to refer back to your mental outline and see what concept, picture, and related information that word is associated with.

For classes that are based on lectures, tape your classes and get copies of notes from other people in your class. Work hard to improve your note taking skills. Take notes on the most important information. If your teacher says something twice, writes it on the board or overhead, or spends extra time on it, it is probably important. Also, read the assigned chapters in your book prior to going to class. That way you will already have an idea of what is going to be discussed.

Another approach that is helpful is studying in a group. Work with a partner or a number of people from your class and study together to prepare for the test. This is something that I try to do a few days before the test. I learn from other people, and they learn from me. The things that they think are important may be things I haven't even thought of and vice versa. I take notes and learn from the study group, then on the last days before the test I find a quiet room and work by myself.

One word of caution about study groups. If they are just a rap session on what everyone is doing over the weekend, they are a waste of time. You would be better off on your own. Find good people, the ones that you would look at in you class and say, "That person really knows their stuff," and get together with them. One important thing to remember is that you need to come to the group prepared. You should have something to contribute. People will look forward to your involvement if you actively participate and share in the group.

If you would prefer not to get help from a group of people, you can very easily and discretely ask someone in your class if they could help you. You would be amazed at the number of people who will help you if you just ask.

After studying the material, one of the most successful ways that I found to prepare for a test was to actually practice taking one. First, I would make a practice test for myself. I would go through my notes and my book, and look for possible questions that might be on the test. Then I would make a practice test for myself by writing out these questions in test form. Another way to do this is to go through the book, look at topic headings, and try to say out loud or write down everything you know about that particular subject. If a teacher gave me a study sheet or possible test questions, I would learn every possible way that test question could be phrased and practice answering those questions. I would always ask for extra study sheets and practice tests if they were given out at school so that I could go home and practice. Also, I found that sometimes there was a study guide that accompanied my text book that had helpful ideas on how to study for the test and had mock tests for specific chapters. A teacher's guide to your text book may also have these things in them.

Knowing the information and being able to recall it in a test situation can often be two different things. Learning disabled students often need to take their tests in a quiet room, or they may need to have some extra time to look over their tests to make corrections. Prior to the day of the first test in your class, ask your teacher or professor if you can come in after school or during their teacher preparation period. Use this time with your teacher to explain that you have problems taking tests. See if you can take the test in a quiet room rather than a noisy one or if you can have a longer testing time so that you can look over your answers before turning in your test. Talk to them about other options such as doing your essay test on computer so that you can run the spell check or taking tests verbally or speaking your essays instead of writing them. Yes, it all sounds a little crazy, but if your writing skills under pressure are lower than your verbal skills, speaking an essay is more likely to get you an A than writing it. Teachers want to see your intelligence. If you know that something works for you, talk to them about the possibility of using that avenue to show your knowledge and skills.

If you feel uncomfortable talking with your teachers about this, sometimes a counselor or resource room teacher can help explain why these things are needed. If you present it in the right way, mainstream teachers may be willing to allow for exceptions. If your teacher refuses to help, you will just have to come to class highly prepared and ready to tune out the noises and focus completely on what you are doing. As with everything else, you will have to develop the skills to take tests. It will seem impossible at first. I can't count the number of times I said, "I can't concentrate," to myself. I had trouble reading tests and understanding what I was reading. I knew the information, but because I had trouble under pressure, I seldom got the information out of my head as easily as I could when I was sitting at home. I learned through each test that I took what to do to help myself to prepare for tests and for the testing situation. You will, too.

Once you have studied for the test and made arrangements with your teacher about how the test will be taken, now you must decide on what to do when the test is in front of you and the panic sets in. First of all, take a deep breath. Second, try this helpful hint. I learned that panic could only take over if I let it. When I first felt a wave of panic, I knew that I had to act quickly. I took a piece of blank paper and wrote down some of the information I had studied before I even looked at the test. Granted, some of that material wouldn't actually be on the test, but it helped me to feel confident that I did know the information. If I looked at the test first and saw something I didn't know, I tended to freeze. If I stayed frozen too long, nothing would come forward. I learned to relax and get control by writing for just a couple of minutes on what the test was about.

Most of all, take your time, read the directions carefully, ask for help if the directions aren't clear, and check to make sure that your "fill in the blanks" sheet is filled out correctly before handing it in.

LEARNING HOW TO GET HELP

I spent a lot of time hiding in class, hoping that I wouldn't be noticed. Often I didn't ask for help because I was afraid of what would happen or what people would think if I needed help. Everyone needs help. It's okay to ask for it. In fact, teachers need you to ask. They can't read minds. Your asking for help, even explaining the areas where you are having trouble, will help them to understand what is troubling you in the class and show them how to help you. Sometimes a teacher will look at kids like us and say, "They are perfectly normal, why don't they participate?" If you explain your situation, the teacher will understand more clearly.

There will always be some teachers who don't understand. As you know, I had several of them. If you ask for help from the first person and he doesn't listen or understand, don't think that everyone will be like that. I found teachers were genuinely willing to help when I asked and when I explained that I was having trouble.

I meet a lot of kids who have created a reputation for themselves with the teachers in their school. Maybe you have had hard times and disagreements with some of your teachers, so you think that nobody would listen or care if you tried to change and get some help for yourself. It's never too late to change and to help other people change their opinion of you.

Maybe you acted out in class and spent a lot of time in the principal's office or in the hall. It gets you out of reading, but you end up without a high school diploma or without an education at all. The student may have to take the first step with a teacher whom he has had friction with. Get someone to go with you if you need some support. Leave your anger somewhere else. If you go in with a bad attitude, you won't make any progress.

Make an appointment to see your teacher when you can be alone and won't be rushed. If you go in and explain when you have your teacher's full attention, things will be a lot clearer. If you are worried that you won't know what to say, write your feelings down in a journal or even in a letter. Take that paper with you when you go to speak to your teacher. If you forget what you want to say, refer back to your notes. If you don't want to go alone, take a teacher or a counselor with you to help you express your ideas and your needs. The changes may be gradual, but taking that first step to explain your differences to someone who doesn't understand will often lead you to a new relationship.

Nothing is one-sided, you have to follow up. You can't just go in and say, "Here are my problems, fix them." Each person has to agree to do his part. Each of you has been jilted. You have had teachers who didn't understand; they have had students who wouldn't accept help or help themselves. The time it takes for trust to develop depends on each person. Do your part and usually that person will do his. Show them that you want their help and that you are willing to meet halfway.

Sometimes a teacher (or someone else for that matter) won't understand. If they don't, and you have done everything within your power to make changes, then you may have to see about another teacher in that subject who would be willing to work with you and the challenges that you have.

Granted, you can't move to another teacher's class at the end of the quarter. The first week would be a good time to make changes if you need to take this route. I had to wait out many a class with a teacher who didn't understand. In time, I learned to observe my teachers and the way they taught so that I would know right away if I could function in that class. I knew I needed structure and step-by-step teaching. Sometimes it was obvious from the start that a teacher did not teach in this way. If that was the only teacher for the subject, then I might be stuck; but if there was a second class being taught by another teacher, then I could possibly transfer in the first week of the quarter or trimester.

Don't quit the class. Find a strategy to stay in it, or get into another teacher's class. Ask your counselor or friends not for the easiest teacher, but for the ones that they liked best. Are they patient? How do they teach? What kind of atmosphere do they allow in the room? Is it noisy or quiet? I learned to ask all the questions before I signed up for the class and it saved me a lot of time and energy.

ALTERNATIVE FORMS OF LEARNING

This whole chapter is about choices and alternatives. There will be some things that worked for me that won't work for you - but some things might. Most of you reading this, no matter what your age or where you are in school, will have to find your own way at times. You will find what type of lighting, background noise, and amount of time spent studying at one sitting is right for you. I am showing you the way I have learned to learn; you add your experiences to the list.

Before I leave this section I want to stress the three things that worked for me in seventh grade and are still working for me today. I use my audio skills. I prefer to hear everything in repetition rather than read it. I use organizational skills to help keep myself organized and on track. And I use the rest of my senses in a multi-sensory way, using constant repetition to fill in the gaps.

There are some learning disabled people who do not have trouble with reading. They can read anything and remember it well. They may want to read their information rather than hear it. I can read, but hearing works best for me.

I guess I have always been an auditory learner. From the time that I could run my record player I would wear the needle out playing my story book records over and over again. The very things I couldn't seem to grasp from a book I could learn from a record, radio, TV, or other audio form.

In seventh grade my sister was trying to help me learn my vocabulary words. She put a word into a tape recorder, then left a space for me to spell it, then she would repeat the word and its spelling. I could learn my vocabulary words much faster this way because I could hear them. Somehow the connection was made. I continued using tape recorders from that time forward.

I still prefer to hear everything that I learn. I tape all of my lectures, and I get books on tape whenever I can. If I can't get my books on tape from a library or book store, then I actually tape them myself or have someone do it for me. Not everyone can tape their own books. I can read out loud with relative ease, I just don't remember a thing that I read. I may not learn anything while reading my chapters onto tape, but once they are on tape, they are my best learning tool. I can then listen to my book on a headset, in my car or on my home stereo.

It only takes a little bit longer to listen to a book on tape than it does to read it. Try it. You might find that it works for you.

At the high school level and especially at the college level I have found tape recorders to be very useful. I carry a small tape recorder to class every day. I tape lectures and even the movies that we have in class. Tape recorders that are made today are so inconspicuous that nobody even notices that I am taping. If I could go back to junior high, I would carry one to all my classes, especially those like history and science classes that have lectures. If it works, use it.

You have already heard my tips on organization. That's how I survived then, and it's how I survive now. I am no longer a scatterbrain. I keep files with everything color coded, and I have date books and organizers to keep my life in order. I write myself notes, keep records of everything, and ask lots of questions about what time something starts and where I am to meet someone, making sure my directions are correct as well as other little details so that I am not late or without the proper materials.

I no longer self-sabotage myself by being late, disorganized, or forgetful. What my mind can't seem to do on it's own, I do for it. Being organized is what sets me apart from the next person. I'm not only organized in school, I am organized in life.

Teachers and parents, start early with your kids. Teach them, remind them, and help them to be organized, and soon they will be able to do it on their own. Kids, it is up to you to take some initiative to help yourself, also. Do everything that you can to become organized both at home and at school and life will be a lot easier for you, your parents, and your teachers.

Using all my senses to the fullest is also what has set me apart and brought me to where I am today. My brain is strange, but I make up for it in effort. I use my eyes to read in repetition, my ears to hear in repetition, my hand to write in repetition, and I use my voice to repeat the information over and over and over again until it makes the connection. I touch it, build it, write it, say it; I do whatever I need to make the information cross the line from misunderstanding to understanding.

Using this "all senses" type of learning, I found out how smart I really was. You would have to be smart to figure out how a brain with learning disabilities works in the first place and then to achieve A's with it! I hope this proves that learning disabled people are intelligent and capable. We just have to find out which path we need to take to find understanding and what type of alternative to use for learning.

I am not telling you that a perfect report card is what makes you a valuable person, but if you want to do better, whatever better is for you, I want you to know that you can improve and will improve. Find a new way - your way.

TEACHERS' TRIBUTES

During the first semester of my seventh grade year, I started to see progress. I worked hard using all of my alternatives. Because of my learning problems, I often had trouble with tests, so I had to do extra credit as well as other work to achieve a high grade. I used every alternative I could find to get the information to make sense, I did extra credit, and most importantly, I received help from several teachers who made the difference in my life. With their help and my determination, I walked out of the first semester with a 4.0 - a straight A report card.

Teachers often get negative attention from the media, and sometimes from the community, too. It saddens me that the focus in our society is on the one teacher who isn't good rather than the millions who are. I would like to share two remarkable teachers who taught me lessons that changed my life forever.

MRS. ELLIS

Mrs. Ellis was dedicated to teaching. Her room was neat, organized and quiet at all times. Her teaching was step by step and as organized as her room. I hadn't been in class like hers since years ago in Miss Driscoll's class. The minute I walked in I thought, "I can make it here."

I had every reason to fear. This was math class, my most feared of all subjects. I was afraid of the subject, but there was something special about Mrs. Ellis. In her class you could tell that she wanted you to learn, and she did everything within her power to make it possible.

Finally, I could concentrate. Everything was organized, and in that environment my brain calmed down and became more organized, too. She used colored assignment sheets which listed assignments as well as the test and quiz dates. This helped me to feel more in control. I knew when the test was coming so I could prepare. I knew what the assignment was going to be the next day so I could read ahead and be prepared when I came to class.

Because her room was quiet during work time, I could do my assignments at school and get help during class. And I was able to understand everything I was hearing. Some people thought she was tough because she held to her classroom rules, but I found her to be a nice, warm person. Her rules made it possible for me to learn.

She never scolded me for asking another question or made me feel intimidated by her knowledge and my lack of it. She saw how much I tried, and she was more than willing to help me or anyone else who needed it.

I achieved my first success in math because of her. The year before I hadn't learned anything, certainly not math skills. The year before that was almost the same. In her class, I was no longer afraid of math. In fact, her way of teaching made it seem interesting and a challenge rather than something to be dreaded.

In her class I learned something that I needed desperately. She was the one who planted the seed that to survive in her class, I would have to become organized. Because of her, I got a hole punch and reinforcers for my papers. I started to take pride in my work, recopying assignments just so that they would look better and be more readable and clear.

I knew that I needed to be organized; but until her class, I had never really thought out how to do that. I watched her; her manner, speech, and actions were easy to follow. Her handouts were clear and easy to read. From the first day on, I not only wanted to please her, I wanted to have that organized quality that she had. Eventually I did, with her help.

I don't know if she had any idea of the impact she made on me; but she cared deeply about everyone in her class, and I was no exception. A couple years ago, I wrote her a letter at Christmas time to thank her for all that she had done. After her class, I had five more years of straight A's in math.

I recently spoke at my old junior high. Mrs. Ellis is still there teaching numbers and equations. Her room is still organized and her kids still love her. Kids like me come back to tell her the difference that she made in their lives, and that keeps her going.

MR. PERCINI

Mr. Percini was funny. He had a certain way about him that made me look up to him, respect him and want to do my best in his class. Sure, I wanted to do well in everyone's class, but his class was like Mrs. Ellis's, you wanted to try that much harder for him than for anyone else.

As with Mrs. Ellis, there were rules in his class, a format and a pattern as to how things would go. You knew what was going to happen, but class was never boring. He was my language arts and social studies teacher. We had spelling tests and all the normal activities in his classroom, but he was creative in his approach to teaching.

We did oral book reports in his class. We would dress up as a main character in the books that we reported on.

I was Maria Vonn Trapp, the heroin in the true life story that the musical, The Sound of Music, was based on. I dressed in a nun's habit and came in singing, "The hills are alive with the sound of music." It was a fun way to learn. He didn't put up with breaking the rules in his class. I respected him for that. He wanted kids to learn and would help us in any way that he could. I learned many things from him but the most important lesson was that cheating cheated yourself.

I wanted to get an A so badly that once on a spelling test when we were supposed to correct another student's paper, I corrected my own and gave myself two words. I had never cheated before. I was always worried about getting in trouble; cheating didn't seem worth it. But the desire to get an A and my difficulty with this particular vocabulary list was so great that I thought, "Well, maybe just this time."

My teacher found out, but he didn't yell at me or make a big fuss. He just told the class that somebody hadn't been honest on the test and he would have to discard the test unless that person came forward. After school, I went in crying. I was never so sorry for having disappointed someone. He forgave me and I promised never to cheat again.

He could have embarrassed me. Instead, he let me realize that cheating was a lie. I was so impressed by him and so embarrassed with myself. I realized that day that keeping an A in any class was not worth cheating. If I did cheat and get an A, then it would be a lie. If I cheated my way though life, my whole life would be a lie. I made the decision then that I didn't want my successes to be lies.

I will thank Mr. Percini for that lesson someday. What an important rule to learn which applies to all aspects of life.

I hope every child will make the decision never to cheat. There are other ways to make it, regardless of our challenges. In a recent interview, Dexter Manley, defensive end for the Washington Redskins, said that he was born with learning problems that have plagued him his whole life. He had to cheat to survive in school. As an adult, he is just now learning to read and is being honest with himself and others about his problems. No grade is worth cheating for. If you tried, even an honest D or F is better than cheating.

You don't have to cheat, that's what this whole chapter is about. Learning disabled people are smart. We can either use our energy and talents to become great cheaters or to be honest with ourselves and find a strategy to learn that will make us successful.

When I graduated from high school, it wasn't a lie. Your life doesn't have to be, either.

CHAPTER 11

To say that I felt great when I looked at my report card would be quite an understatement. What could I tell you that would help you to understand the kind of high that it gave me to see those A's? To be at the top of the class rather than at the bottom had been only a dream before, now it was reality. My family thought it was wonderful, but only my mom could truly know what this meant to me. Only she knew how great the odds were against my ever achieving straight A's.

It was possible. It did happen. Now what? I became determined to keep my A's. They became my ticket to a better life, and I was now one of the mainstream. No one could deny me. I started a new quarter convinced that now I would have everything that I had always wanted. People would like me, my father would be proud. The past would finally be behind me.

I hope that you can hear from these last sentences that the grades were not achieved just for my satisfaction. As much as I wanted to say it was for me, my self-image was dependent upon trying to please everyone around me. In part, my grades were earned for all of the people whom I wanted to please - all those who had said I was not smart enough. In doing this, I was giving away the joy of my accomplishment.

I proved this when I took my report card down to my elementary school and walked into my former 6th grade classroom to find my teacher. He had become the symbol of all those who didn't believe in me. I guess I thought that if I took my report card and showed it to him, he would be moved to change his mind about me. I thought he would say, "Shari, I was so wrong about you; you are smart."

He didn't even look up when I came into the room. Finally I said, "Hello."

He said, "Hello," and continued on with his work. After some small talk, I held up my report card. He looked at it and went back to his work with no pat on the back, nothing. What was it that I expected him to do? He was what he was. No more, no less. He didn't have praise for me when I was a student in his class, why would he have any now? But he stood as the symbol. He was my father, my past teachers, the friends, the relatives. I felt that if he could tell me I was smart enough and good enough, somehow it would make up for the past. But he was a person who didn't want to be teaching. I can safely say now that he didn't really care about me. So what was I doing there?

Maybe I already knew this would happen, but the need for praise was so great that I would put myself in a vulnerable position again and again. Always trying to show that I was good enough to be liked. Always begging for praise, often from those who wouldn't give it to me even if they could. It is a tiring process, always trying to prove yourself, never feeling good enough for other people or yourself.

I was suffering from this lack of praise. I got the grades and achieved, but was it for all the wrong reasons? When all the dust cleared, I was left standing with nothing to call my own. The dream belonged to those who said, "You never will be successful." I handed them my pride and accomplishments, and at any time they could change the rules or the line that I must cross to receive their acceptance. It would be years before my dreams, goals, and hopes were truly my own. Then, I lived with the false sense that I was doing it all for me, an exhausting journey to nowhere. Yes, I had the grades, but what else? When you don't believe in yourself, you have very little.

When reality sunk in a few weeks later, I realized that to maintain my grades I would have to work as hard I had before. I could never let up. The reward seemed to be worth it. I didn't spend a lot of time with friends or have any outside activities, so that left plenty of time to devote to school. I continued with the late nights and early mornings and found myself looking forward to summer and a rest for my brain.

I didn't have many friends, but having good grades and achieving my long-awaited goal seemed to curb my loneliness. Most friendships that I did have were short lived. These friends had more money, bigger houses, and more affluent parents. I was told that the only reason I had any friends at all was because my sister was a cheerleader. It hurt me, but I knew they were right.

People knew me because I had a beautiful, popular sister at school. I was known only as Shawn's little sister most of the year, but I didn't mind. I was extremely proud of her. I followed her, mimicked her, and longed to be all the things that she was. I started to understand what it was like for Jennifer the year before.

Jennifer was like me, the loner, the outcast. With Shawn around, people knew her name. She had someone to eat lunch with, she had a new group of friends. Probably for the first time in her life, Jennifer was not alone. I started to feel the same way.

Without Shawn at that school, I don't know what it would have been like for me. Even with her there, I found myself standing on the outside looking in at the girls who were supposed to be my friends. These were the girls of the sixth grade wing. The ones who had shut me out the year before because I wasn't like them. Now, with a new pair of contact lenses and a popular sister, all of a sudden I can stand next to them in the lunch line, just not too close. While things were not the best, they were certainly better than before. Whether it was due to my sister or not, I rode the crest of semi-popularity and enjoyed it while it lasted.

While my life was starting over, Jennifer's life was in a tailspin.

She was now alone up at the high school, searching to find friends who would accept her, searching for love. Few people saw her. Now she no longer had someone to eat lunch with nor did she have the gossip of the day to discuss with Shawn when they both returned home from school. These had been important moments to her.

She had gained self-esteem the year before and had lost weight. Now she was back sliding. We were so much alike. The difference was that by seventh grade things were changing for me. She, on the other hand, had few successes, she hadn't found her way yet. Yes, we were a lot alike, except for one thing. She killed herself at age fifteen.

I would love to think that it was some mistake, that she was just trying to get our attention; but we will never know that for sure. Suicide is not reversible. You can't take it back if it goes too far. That's why I speak of my stepsister now. I hope that others will learn through Jennifer's story that suicide is not a way out. Living is the only real choice. If Jennifer was trying to get attention, she was playing Russian Roulette with all of our lives and with our love for her. I feel regret for the life that she will never lead and for our lost relationship.

The circumstances surrounding Jennifer's death are not something I choose to elaborate on. You can't bring the dead back by pointing the finger at one person or laying the blame on one situation. It is never that simple. Although there may be one final blow that will push someone over the edge into a suicide attempt, it isn't usually one thing that leads to depression and ultimately suicide.

I write about Jennifer's death without blame. I write about her with hope, hope that others will read this and think twice before choosing suicide as their solution. I write with thanks for the understanding I gained through losing her. Because of her death, I learned to live and to cherish life.

SUICIDE

One day after school, we were stopped by one of my sister's friends. She told us that my mom didn't want us to take the bus home but wanted us to go over to her house for awhile and we would be picked up there. That didn't sound so out of the ordinary to my sister or me, and we did it without question. Everyone seemed to be in good spirits when we arrived at her house, but when we asked why my mom couldn't pick us up, everyone tried to change the subject. As time went on, things started to feel very strange. Then the phone rang. It was my mom. She talked to my sister and then to me. She said Jennifer was hurt and in the hospital. Before my mom hung up the phone, she told my sister that Jennifer had tried to commit suicide by hanging herself in our garage. We were told to go to a friend's house because she didn't want us to come home and see the ambulance parked out in front of our home.

I couldn't even cry because it didn't seem real. Jennifer was alive and in the hospital. I just kept thinking, she is alive and will be all right; she is in a coma but she is alive.

She lived for a week. That week stands out in my mind as some kind of bizarre nightmare with everything moving in slow motion, with no feeling being completely real.

It was a cold, ugly week. As ugly outside as I felt inside. I went to school wondering who would understand this mess. Certainly not my "friends." I decided that Jennifer had to get better, then no one would have to know. I would just go on pretending that everything was okay. Just as I had learned to cover my differences, I handled this situation the same way. If others didn't know, I wouldn't have to explain. I couldn't have explained anyway, I didn't understand it myself. How could someone do this?

That theory would have worked if people's curiosity hadn't gotten the best of them. From the day after Jennifer attempted suicide, gossip began spreading throughout the school like a plague. It started with a girl named Darcy who lived across the street from us. She had heard the ambulance at our house and came across the street to see what had happened.

Prior to this time, Darcy had been such a shy girl. She wasn't shy any longer. By the time I got to school the next day, everyone knew. It never occurred to me that it was Darcy who had told everyone until I reached my chorus class. She came up to me and started asking detailed questions about what had happened, expecting me to tell her. During class, I heard her whispering in the ears of the surrounding students. I couldn't believe her nerve. I realize now that she may not have known any better, but I found it hard to believe that someone would find it so interesting to discuss something so awful.

One of the girls sitting next to me asked, "Shari, what happened?" She was a friend so I thought that it was better if she finds out from me instead of from someone else. I tried to tell her, but the words just got stuck. Everyone was shuffling and preparing their music, some were laughing and joking with each other; and there I was, trying to tell someone that my sister was in the hospital dying. My head started to pound and tears started to fall. I had never walked out of a class before, but I headed right for the door. The room became silent as the door shut behind me.

The first person I thought of was my sister, Shawn. Shawn would understand, I needed to find her. I ran across the walkway to the gym. The air was cold, but I could hardly feel it as I ran to the locker room. Normally I would have felt self-conscious, wondering what people would think of me with my tear-stained face and red nose. Not now. This time, it didn't seem to matter what other people thought, I was in too much pain to think about it.

My sister knew why I was there. She put her arm around me and we walked out of the gym and into the locker room. We talked and cried, both of us feeling helpless and confused. Seeing her made me feel better. She was the rock to me, even when she cried. I still felt she was stronger than me.

After I put myself together again, we hugged each other and I went back to my class as the bell was ringing. I didn't want to face anybody, so I waited until I thought the room was clear and I went in to get my books.

The room still had a few people in it when I entered. One of them was a boy who was an acquaintance of mine. We didn't really know each other very well, certainly not well enough to talk about this. He stopped me when I entered the room and asked what was wrong. I told him and started to cry some more. He tried to understand, though I didn't expect him to.

After he left, I gathered up my books and apologized to my teacher for leaving. He said, "Shari, there's nothing to worry about. I'm sorry about Jennifer. I had her as a student when she was in junior high."

He asked me how she was and I said, "Not very well." He shook his head and I left.

I finished that day and tried to get through the next. Each day, Jennifer became worse. The doctors were saying that she would probably never come out of her coma. I still kept believing that she would come home, that a miracle would happen and this would all be over.

Thursday of that week when Mom returned from the hospital, she told me that it looked like Jennifer was going to die. I was standing in our living room leaning up against the couch, looking into the big mirror we had hanging on the wall.

I remember that I was blow drying my hair. I know that may seem like a strange place to be styling my hair, but it had become part of our morning ritual. Shawn, Jennifer, and I would line up in front of the big mirror and do our hair every morning. There was a small transistor radio hidden under the skirt of a nearby table, and we would congregate at the mirror with our makeup and curling irons. They would pick the radio station which I would groan about, and then they would look at each other and roll their eyes. That's how every day had begun.

On that particular morning, I was alone at the mirror and, surprisingly enough, was feeling rather optimistic. Something kept telling me that at any moment, someone was going to say, "It's a mistake; it was all a dream. Jennifer isn't sick, she's just away

177

on a trip." I hadn't been allowed to see her yet, the hospital, the bed. It seemed unreal.

My mom told me that Jennifer was dying and there was little hope for recovery. I looked at my mom and it still didn't hit me. The only thing in my life that had ever died was my hamster, Pete, and a favorite cat. I couldn't understand what it meant to have a person die. I knew then that I had to see her if she wasn't going to live. I had to touch her and say good-bye.

Everyone had kept us from seeing her in the hospital. Everybody thought it would be better for us not to see her as she was then, but to remember her alive and well. But there was something strong telling me I had to go see her.

That night we were allowed to go to the hospital. Jennifer was in a room with other coma victims. We stayed in the waiting room outside until the nurses said we could all go in.

I had no idea what to expect; my legs felt wobbly, but I knew this was my chance. I thought maybe it would turn out as it does in the movies where if you talk to the person long enough, she will connect with your voice and come out of the coma. If you say, "I love you," and hold her hand, she will open her eyes and come back to you. I guess that's what I thought we were going to do. At first, I went to see her because I wanted to say good-bye. Now, I thought maybe I could bring her back, I could will her back to life if I could just get in there to see her.

I walked into a room filled with sleeping people; bed after bed of motionless people, some young, and some old. When I think back on the scene, all the other people in the room seemed to have been in the shadows. Their beds, blankets, and even their faces were sort of grey and hazy. Then I saw her. She was white, like white light, not grey like everyone else. Her face was shiny and clean with her hair pulled back with a ribbon. She looked so beautiful and peaceful, it seemed that I could hear what her laughter had sounded like.

Bob stood holding her hand and he kept squeezing it three times to symbolize "I love you." He gave me her hand and I tried it. He said he was waiting for her to squeeze back. She never did.

Tears came hard as I watched her sleeping. "I can save her, I can save her," I kept thinking to myself. "If I stand here long enough, I can save her. If I stroke her hair, she will come back to life." But it was too late. They wanted to take me out of the room but I wouldn't go. "I can save her, just a little bit longer. Don't make me go," I pleaded. I knew when I entered the room that it might be the last time I would see her. I kept thinking, "If I stay, she won't die; as long as I stay here, there is a chance."

They took me out of the room, sobbing and begging to stay by her side. The next morning she was gone.

The next day I went to school early to finish an assignment I had to hand in. I had worked a week ahead in my studies because my dad had planned a trip to Hawaii for Shawn and me. Having a large amount of work to do may have kept my mind busy during our week of tragedy, but that morning I felt numb and tired.

It is amazing to me that our trip happened to come just three days after my stepsister died. I didn't really want to go because of everything that had happened. I couldn't think of enjoying myself in Hawaii knowing that Jennifer had just died. My mom felt it was best if we went while she and Bob took Jennifer to the family burial site. She felt it would be better for us not to go with them or to stay at home alone.

So there I was, finishing my last assignment in math so I wouldn't fall behind when I got back. Mrs. Ellis, my math teacher, raised her head from her desk and looked at me saying, "Shari, I'm sorry to hear about Jennifer. Is she doing any better?"

At that moment, I saw that same image of Jennifer in that room of grey people, out of all of them, she was the white light. I saw her as clear as day, then I had to say what I knew was true. I said, "No, she passed away," and I began to cry.

In the days that followed, most people seemed either to say something out of line or nothing at all. It was as if they feared saying anything out loud about suicide, or someone who committed suicide, because it might happen to them. The curious onlookers watched and made their assessments. Some were even bold enough to ask questions that were none of their business, but nobody seemed to care that we felt dead inside and that their careless remarks were stabbing me like a knife.

There was this great need to talk, and cry and get it out; but I was so afraid of what people would think if I did. I held it all inside out of fear of rejection.

The media has begun dealing with the subject of death and has also addressed the high rates of suicide across our country, especially among young people. There are more after-school specials, documentaries, and other parent, teacher, and student information resources then ever before. Thanks to this media effort, the word suicide is no longer a word that you whisper in private. I support the changes that are taking place in our schools and communities and in society in general. These changes help to shed some light on a long covered up topic.

When I was in school, though, there were no such programs. People rarely mentioned death of natural causes or accidents, let alone mention a death as undignified as taking your own life. There was so much ignorance; even I didn't understand what suicide meant. I thought only crazy, insane people killed themselves. Kamakazi pilots and people jumping off buildings during the stock

179

market crash; those were my references. People who were crazed committed suicide, not normal people.

Death makes people feel so vulnerable. It seems that someone made a rule that if you don't talk about, it doesn't exist. We tried that with drugs, teenage pregnancy, and divorce. We didn't talk about those issues until the problems were out of control; then we were forced to deal with them. When you can't talk about your problems or your feelings, you feel isolated and alone. I was sure no one had ever gone through what I was going through. I write and speak about this now because it is important to me that no one should ever feel as alone as I did after Jennifer's death.

We do know more now, but we need to continue to encourage people to make the choice to live. Jennifer's problems didn't go away by ignoring them or pretending they weren't there. No, they didn't go away, she went away. We can't wait to hear the cries for help or other people will go away, too.

A few weeks after Jennifer's death, it was over for those who hadn't been close to her. For the rest of us, it would never be over.

I guess that is the irony of suicide. Some people kill themselves to make others feel sorry or to make someone miss them. Some people have said after surviving a suicide attempt that what they really wanted - their greatest fantasy after they died - was to imagine themselves looking down, watching people mourn, particularly those who hurt them at one point or another.

What ends up happening is that their death affects most cruelly the ones who loved them the most, not the ones who didn't. They might have killed themselves to get back at someone, maybe they had a fight, or any number of things that causes them to say, "I'll make that person sorry." When they do it, they may not want to hurt friends, teachers, or relatives, but none of these people go unscathed.

People who were close to the victim will be drained by the pain and frustration of the death. Sometimes people are never the same after a suicide; family members don't speak to each other and they blame each other. Those who didn't truly care will just go on with their lives.

Instead of just mourning, those who feel the loss of the suicide get angry and frustrated. They feel badly for getting angry because the person they love is dead. They feel guilt and worry, thinking about all the things they should have done or could have said to save that person. The truth is, the aftermath of a suicide and its effects on people is never the fantasy that people imagine.

What do you do when people just start to go on with their lives, but you are still filled with pain? What happens to the loved ones who are left behind? What happens when you need to cry, but no one wants to hear it? It makes others uncomfortable, they would rather not deal with the pain because it makes them feel helpless; they don't want to get near you because they might catch it.

What do you do when you go home to a house filled with sadness? There are memories everywhere, but few people who understand. You learn to get through it in whatever way that you can. That's what you do.

My sister and I left for Hawaii as planned. I don't think that we talked about her death even once the whole time we were gone, we were so numb. Looking back, I know that getting away was probably good for both of us, and yet it made coming home even more painful. Nothing had healed; it couldn't heal in only a week. No answers could be found. We came home to a house heavy with pain; all we had done was delay the painful process of recovering from this tragedy.

CHOOSING HOW TO SAY GOOD-BYE

While we were gone, Jennifer was buried. Even if we had been home, I don't think my mom would have allowed us to go to the funeral. We had said our good-byes at the hospital.

But we did attend Jennifer's memorial service. I did not want to go. It was held two weeks after her death and we were just beginning to get a grip on ourselves. Having a memorial service re-opened every wound.

People got up during the service and talked about how they knew Jennifer. What could anybody say now that could take away her pain? I couldn't help but think how strange it was that we were coming together to say nice things about someone who was dead, someone who felt so badly about herself that she took her own life in desperation. If only these things could have been said to her when she was alive, maybe she would still be here. I felt angry at everyone, including myself. "We didn't do enough for Jennifer!," I wanted to shout. But I kept it in - once again, I kept it in.

That memorial service didn't heal me in any way. To the contrary, it filled me with anger and regrets. I didn't know who to blame, so I blamed myself. I needed an answer, so I decided that I should have been there more for her. I knew there were other reasons she took her life, but none of them were clear. Just like with my parents' divorce, I assumed there must have been something more that I could have done.

Following the memorial service, we had to perform what seemed like a very strange ritual. This ritual involved having everyone from the service come over to our house to have refreshments and visit. Granted, I knew this was customary, but all I wanted was to hide somewhere away from people, questions, and thoughts. I didn't want people coming over to our house, wandering around

181

and saying how sorry they were one more time. I didn't want them to invade my memory and thoughts with their stories of how they knew her and the good times they had. How could they talk and carry on? All I could feel was numbness, and their laughter made me hate them all.

If you want to know what a kid thinks about a situation like this, here is Shari Rusch at age thirteen on the death of her stepsister: Stop, world. Stop everything. Don't laugh. Just give respect. Don't forget her. Don't gossip or laugh about the past. Don't invade this house with your laughter, your drinking, your eating, and your kind gestures. Just make her come back. Can you do that? No? Well then, just leave and let me sort this out. You didn't save her, so leave. I couldn't save her, so leave me alone. I can't sleep because I see her. I can't live in this house because she lived here. I can't talk about it because there are no answers. All of you people can leave, but I have to walk by her bedroom every day to get to the bathroom. I sit at the table every night and do my homework by the garage where she hung herself. No kind word could fix that. No memorial service could fix that. No pasta salad get together afterwards could fix that.

Towards the end of the day, a song that was popular at the time came on the radio. It was a song called "Dog and Butterfly." It was a song Jennifer loved, and listening to it reminded me of her. I remember listening to it that day and telling one of her school friends who was sitting next to me to listen to the words - they were just like Jennifer. The song talks about a dog and butterfly, and about how the dog would like to fly up in the air with the butterfly, but she can't and she falls back down on the ground.

Jennifer was innocent, wanting to fly, but reality kept holding her to the ground, to the harshness of life. When she was running and laughing with her dog, she was free. In her writings she talked about animals, cats, dogs, and maybe even a butterfly or two. These are the "Dog and the Butterfly" memories of Jennifer. I wish she could have flown longer while she was on earth. I pray now that she is in a place where she is free to fly like a butterfly.

□

For many years I feared that someone I loved would die. I didn't feel that I would have the strength to go through the process of grieving that I had experienced when we lost Jennifer. Death was a dark ugly tunnel because my only knowledge of death was from the act of suicide. I see things differently now.

I recently lost my grandfather and yes, it was painful to lose someone I loved. But the truth is, I was able to tell him that I loved him. I was there with him in the hospital before he died. I saw a dignity in him that was so profound I cannot find the words to describe it. He was eighty years old. He and my grandmother had fifty-five wonderful years together, and he had greatly influenced my life and the lives of many others in his lifetime.

Losing him made me realize the need for the memorial service, the funeral and all the other things that I saw as just awkward rituals before. Each of these customs is about honoring not the death, but the life of a great human being.

Death is no longer frightening to me. It is a dignified passage to heaven and all the rewards that wait there.

A MESSAGE TO THE SURVIVORS

When I was little and I fell down and skinned my knee at recess, I'd cry a little but could make it through the rest of the day. As soon as I hit our yard and saw my mom, my injured knee would start hurting again and the tears would come running down my face. What had been a simple scratch would now feel like an emergency-room catastrophe.

In elementary school it's a skinned knee; by junior high and high school the problems get bigger. But not all moms and dads are there for you when you need some attention or need to talk. You come home from school with the weight of the world on your shoulders and need to talk to someone that cares; but there isn't anybody there.

For most kids, that somebody isn't going to get home until six o'clock at night when they return home from work. Then when they do get home, time is filled with preparing dinner, doing housework, and washing dishes. By that time, kids have hidden their pain to keep from disrupting the schedule, handled it on their own, or feel that there is no one to share it with. That is a conventional family; a family where the parents come home at a reasonable time and are even open to sharing with their children.

It's nice to have two parents coming home at night, but that isn't the norm anymore. The norm is one parent, overwhelmed, working full time to make ends meet. Kids are coming home from school and living on their own in the afternoons with little or no supervision. What do you do with your hurt until your mom or dad gets home? Even more important, what do you do if you can't talk to your parents, if every conversation ends in a shouting match? What do you do if your parents are the source of your pain? What do you do in a family riddled with alcoholism? You learn not to come home. You learn to find a way to deal with your problems on your own, which often means drugs, alcohol, and other destructive escapes.

What do you do when you are the "adult" in the house for several hours a day, taking care of your brothers and sisters and you are hurting about something? Where do you go with your pain?

Fortunately, when I was growing up, I always had my mom's work telephone number. I knew that I could call at any time, and that made me feel secure. I was a loner and hid my feelings inside. I found it hard to share my pain with anyone besides my mother because I felt that no one would understand. If I could hold my tears in until I got home, I could call my mom and talk it out with her. I had a lifeline; I had someone to go to. Many kids do not have that luxury.

The day my stepsister attempted suicide, everything was crashing around her. She was not doing well at school; in fact, she had flunked several tests in a row in the same class. She had a disagreement with her father and was alone in the house for an hour before the rest of the family came home from school and work. My mom called her from work and knew that Jennifer was hurting. She said, "Jennifer can you hold on until I can get there?" Jennifer didn't answer. My mom raced through traffic to get home, knowing in the back of her mind that Jennifer might try to take her life. She thought she could get there in time, but when she got home, it was too late.

As Jennifer lay in a coma in the intensive care unit in the hospital, one of the nurses said that the hours between three and five p.m. and night time are the worst hours of the day for suicide. It is a time when kids are alone with their problems. Maybe they can't or won't call their parents at work or even worse, maybe their parents are part of the problem. The kid waits through the afternoon with the paper with the F on it, the note from school that has to be signed, or the rejection letter from a boyfriend or girlfriend. The television drones on or the music on the radio describes a lost love, and it fills their minds. They become more lonely and despondent.

Can you wait twenty minutes for someone to get out of freeway traffic? Can you wait until morning when the sun shines again and you can find someone to talk to? Can you wake someone up, can you call a friend, can you wait until you get to school to talk to a counselor? Can you take the time to pick up a phone book and look for a social service agency that has free counselling or an emergency hot line? Can you hold on just a little bit longer? Isn't your life worth holding on for just a little bit longer?

After Jennifer's death, we were all left wondering if she really meant to do it? Did she want my mom to save her? Did she want her father to feel badly because they had an argument over the phone? She left clues that indicated she thought my mom would get to her sooner and be able to save her life as she had before. It was not my mom's fault that there was a traffic jam; it was Jennifer's choice to tempt fate.

Do you see what I am saying? My mom could have helped if Jennifer had waited. They could have talked it out and dealt with the problem. Once Jennifer went to the brink of death it was too late. She will never realize that the fight with her father was not as bad as she thought and that no problem at school was worth her life. None of us will ever know the things that she could have been, the lives she would have influenced for the good, the friends, the activities, the great life she would have led had she lived. If you kill yourself now, you will never know either.

Robert Schuller calls suicide a "permanent solution to a temporary problem." You can't take it back; force yourself to hold on. The thing that is painful now may be less so by tomorrow. It won't last forever, you must remember that. Remind yourself of that when you start thinking that the only way out is death. If you can't talk to your family or they aren't available, find anybody you can trust, anybody who is available and will listen. But know this: they can listen, they can help, they can "will" you to live like my mom previously did for Jennifer. But nobody can truly help you unless you make the decision to live.

When no one else is around you must will yourself to live. In the long run there will not always be someone around to save you. There will not always be that encouraging voice to cheer you on. At some point, we all must make the decision to live. We must be that little voice inside saying, "Don't give up." We cannot always save someone else. As much as we would like to, few people can make someone else live. I cannot make you live. I can help you, love you, and listen; I can even beg you, but eventually the choice becomes yours.

When I was afraid and alone and felt there was no one to turn to, I prayed. The simplest of prayers would do. There is a power greater than you. If you have no one to turn to here on earth, don't give up. You are not alone. I wouldn't have believed it myself until I saw God work in my life throughout my loneliest times. The first step is asking for help.

As teachers and parents, we must look for the requests for help and acknowledge them as real. The passing comment, the skipping of class, the dull, lifeless eyes, the listless unresponsiveness in kids. Sometimes the signs are hard to detect, but if you are open and encourage students to talk about their problems on a one-to-one basis, they may come to you rather than trying to handle it by themselves.

They will not snap out of it; it is not a just a phase that they are going through. Thoughts of suicide are real and must be addressed as such. I think as soon as adults address the issue for what it is rather than trivialize it as a teenage bout with the blues, then kids will no longer trivialize it as a possible solution or a nice fantasy.

As parents, we must know that success in business can be very rewarding, but the money you earn can't bring back a child who couldn't wait until your business meeting was over to discuss an important problem. Time, although short, is the most important commodity to anybody, especially a struggling child. Listen to what your child is saying, make yourself available, then you won't be picking up the pieces from suicide. No, none of this will save them all, but it is a start.

Teachers, parents, and community members must realize the need for classes teaching coping skills and strategies for dealing with life challenges for our children. We are a nation with a fifty percent divorce rate and latch key children; therefore, we must help kids to develop their abilities to cope with stress and problems. If we don't, we will be losing some of the brightest kids who could have been leading this country in the future. It is not just learning disabled children or children from low income housing, no single race or religion is prone to commit suicide - the victims come from all walks of life. It is proper coping skills and having people available to help children with problems that can make a difference.

I was shocked into reality when my stepsister died. The death was magnified and the pain increased when I didn't have anyone to go to for help. I want other people to see the real side of suicide and be shocked into reality. The most significant thing that came from her death was the fact that I swore from that time forward, I didn't want to have the same thing happen to me. Because I was like her in many ways, I was afraid that maybe it could happen to me. It never did because suicide doesn't just happen to you, it is a choice. Just because your mother or father, sister or brother chose to die, doesn't mean you will.

I am sending a challenge out to all of you to live. Work through your problems and live. It will be worth it to you. This is my message to the surviving, to those who are staying alive right now despite the problems they are going through, and to those who are choosing the courageous way rather than the quick way out.

I am a survivor of suicide. I was one of the people left behind, trying to put together the pieces of a tragedy. I know there are many others like myself and my family. Maybe you are dealing with the loss of a loved one or friend right now. I know what you are going through and it is, without doubt, one of the most difficult things to get through; but you will get through it. Hopefully, you will be able to help someone else in the future with the knowledge that this experience has brought to you, and you will help them with their pain. I hope this message will help you with yours.

Know that it is not your fault. You cannot take responsibility for a choice made by someone else; we each make our own choices. If someone wants to die badly enough, they will find a way. They realize that they need help fast, but may decide life just isn't worth the effort. Once again, that is their choice.

When looking for the source of their pain, explore all the options. Go from the smallest, a problem at school, to the biggest, a hormone imbalance or clinical depression. Seek help from professionals, but always get a second opinion. Talk to everyone including the person who is suicidal, and indicate to them that you are willing to help. Show the possible solutions to their problems and help in whatever way possible to encourage them to seek help for themselves through the school counselor or a professional counselor.

There are limits to what you can do, especially if you are a friend rather than a family member. If the burden is too heavy and someone is leaning on you as their only reason to live, you must shift the weight to other supporters. People who threaten you saying, "If you don't love me, I'm going to die," need more than your shoulders. They need help in ways you can't provide or shouldn't have to provide. Let others know of the problem. When people think you are the only one who knows, it becomes a nice little secret or possibly even a ploy to get your attention. When you tell someone else, it lowers the pressure on you and gets someone else into the picture who can help. I am not saying that a suicidal person is faking it for attention, I am just saying that we don't always know the reasons why someone would threaten a suicide. Let others help you to deal with the problem.

I think it is important not only to take the person at risk seriously and to get them help, but it is also important to turn over the responsibility to that person at some point. You must tell them, "I love you," but let them know that they have to decide to live. Get help for them, love them, but let them know that they have responsibility, too.

If someone you love does choose suicide, it is very hard to know what to do with all the pent up anger and emotion you have inside. Let it out, talk to someone and seek help right away. The longer you wait, the more it will fester and grow. Face the pain and the hurt will heal; run from it and you will just prolong the pain.

Surround yourself with those who will let you feel the pain and get out all the tears that need to be cried. Tears are healthy and cleanse the hurt. There will be some who feel that emotion is messy and will want you to forget about it and snap out of it. Allow yourself to grieve and then get on with your life.

Sometimes you may need to cry about what has happened even after many years have passed. That's okay; those feelings are there for a reason. Experience them instead of covering them up. Crying is a part of the healing process. I covered up my tears for six years, then had to deal with multiples of tears. Cry now.

I would like to suggest that there are self-help groups and counselling groups that may help you to get in touch with what you are feeling, and put you in touch with others who have lost family members or friends through suicide. You may not have someone to talk to who understands, so a group like this may be the right thing for you.

In saying this, I would also like to point out that there are many good support groups, but there are also groups that are nothing but groups of sad people. If you go to a group and come out feeling worse and with fewer answers than when you went in, I suggest you not go again. The same thing is true with a therapist. If you question their methods and practices, find someone else.

I was once invited to speak at what was termed a "Suicide Prevention Banquet." What I ultimately found out was that it was a banquet which would be attended by family members of suicide victims, like a memorial for the dead. There was going to be a rose on each table for each family member or friend who had died. I was shocked when I found out what this banquet was really about and called the director to withdraw my services.

I will not participate in any activity that is locked into the past. To sit around mourning the passing of a loved one by suicide is not constructive; that person is gone. Celebrate the life you have and use their memory for good. Help others, through constructive means, to live. Don't get caught up in anything that will only extend your grief rather than heal it. I told the person in charge, "I am dedicated to life. My hours will be spent changing lives for the better, not giving time to more pain."

Clinging to the past is a sure way to keep you from having a future. I did that for a while, hoping if I just stayed where I was, nothing bad would ever happen again. Instead, I didn't go forward and I didn't lose any of the pain.

Sometimes your subconscious mind will work on things when you're asleep. If you are still harboring pain, guilt, and anger, but you don't deal with it during the day, you may have nightmares at night. Somewhere the feelings exist but haven't been handled. I suffered this kind of nightmare for years before I went for counselling. With counselling, the feelings came out. I didn't have to run from them in my subconscious or conscious mind anymore, and the nightmares went away. Seeking therapy to help work through your pain is courageous, not weak.

Allow yourself to be angry at the person for leaving you. When someone commits suicide, there are unanswered questions, guilt, and loneliness. If this was your best friend, father, mother, sister, or brother, there is so much you wish to share with them, to understand about them; and none of that can be done. Since the person is dead, you feel guilty for getting angry, but if you don't direct your anger towards that person, you take it out on other people or yourself.

Suicide is a very selfish act. The victims think only of what a relief it would be for them. Yet look at what they left behind for those who loved them - a trail of pain. Place the blame where it belongs, the person who took her life must be held responsible for the action. Shout at the ceiling, yell at a picture. Do whatever you have to do to put the anger where it belongs. Rather than blaming yourself, ask, "If that person really cared about me, why would they want to leave me with such pain?" You can still love that person and be angry. You can still miss that person but be angry with the decision that she made.

When we lack answers, we find it easy to blame ourselves. We may never have the answers! If you blame yourself as I did, you can spend the rest of your life feeling guilty. The suicide will just continue to live on unless you forgive yourself. As soon as you give that person credit for the part they had in their own death, the faster your healing.

Feel sorry for yourself, too. Your are as much a victim of the suicide as the one who dies. The difference is that you didn't have a choice in it, your life was affected because of that person's choice. Get realistic, it takes more courage to stay on this earth than it does to check out. You can feel badly about what happened, but remember who did what.

Find outlets that help you vent some of the pain, but make those outlets creative rather than destructive. In the midst of your pain and anger, you may find yourself becoming self-destructive. Don't self-destruct just because someone else did. You may want to just keep sleeping, drinking, or eating to get rid of the pain. Instead, try dance, art, running, self-help books, anything that will remove you from the pain and get the anger out. Volunteer to work at a Ronald McDonald House, a retirement center or a shelter for the homeless. You will be surprised how seeing children with cancer or serving food to those in need will bring your pain into perspective.

When people die, the people left behind tend to want to complete the life that is no longer there, to live out the unfulfilled dreams of the person. But when that person decided she didn't want to live anymore, she also decided that she didn't want to dream anymore. Carry out your purpose in life, not someone else's broken dreams. You cannot recreate or live for that person after they are gone. Make your own dreams come true. Losing someone taught me not to harbor regrets and to say what I wanted to say to the people I love now rather than later. None of us know how long we will be here. Let the disagreements and friction go, forgive others and don't waste your time harboring bad feelings. Say what you want to say today; tomorrow might be too late.

If you are feeling alone and contemplating suicide or living with the aftermath of a suicidal death, look to God for strength, surround yourself with friends and family who love you and support you, and find a supportive counselor who can help.

STUMBLING BLOCKS TO STEPPING STONES

CHAPTER 12

AFTERSHOCK

When Jennifer died, I could feel the poison inside our house. We tried to carry on in spite of the memories; but there was the garage where she had killed herself, and there was her room downstairs by the laundry room. She was everywhere, but nowhere. We couldn't get away from her or our feeling of loss. There wasn't anywhere to go to escape.

There was nothing noble or honorable about Jennifer's death and that's what made it so hard to get over. She had chosen to leave us.

Others went on with their lives and weren't aware of what we were going through; some didn't want to know. You sense this after a tragic death. People don't want to get too close for fear they will catch it like a disease. Seeing tragedy makes them feel vulnerable, so they don't want to get too near the crazy family, the sad tragic family that is falling apart.

What do people think of a family like ours? Do they think we are bad and drove her to her death, that something strange was happening behind closed doors? At thirteen, I worried about what other people thought, and I felt ostracized.

I went to school, pretending that I was the same as before, trying to show everyone that my family was not crazy. I carried on as if to say to everyone, "I am okay. See, I'm not crying anymore. Please still be my friend. I won't talk about it. You won't even know that it happened." I tried to make up for all the bad things I thought people would say about Jennifer by pretending that everything was fine.

Deep down inside I felt that I was a lot like Jennifer. If I started to fail again at school, if I hit rock bottom like she did, would I do the same thing? People often ask what my motivation was for sustaining the kind of grades I did over such a long period of time with the kind of learning problems I had. You just heard it. Jennifer's death would overshadow everything in my life from that time forward.

Sometimes I didn't realize what it was that was driving me so hard, yet it was always there. The truth is, I was scared that if I wasn't perfect enough, people would shut me out, leave me as my stepsister had, and then I would kill myself. The thought was so horrible and ugly, I ran from it. Ran, studied till all hours, didn't go to sleep until I was totally exhausted, did anything to keep from facing the true source of my marathon.

I know now that I wouldn't have killed myself. But at the time, there were no guarantees. My life was upside down. There was no sense to it anymore. People at school were asking bizarre things of us, and life at home was even more bizarre. I asked myself every day, "How did we get into this mess?" Even worse, I kept wondering how we were going to get out of it.

193

LIVING WITH SHADOWS

We had to continue to live every day in a house filled with ghosts. I had never believed in ghosts, but after Jennifer's death, I felt like there were images around corners, hiding in the shadows. They were there, I could feel them. They were her. Not the Jennifer I used to know, but a darker spirit of her.

My mom has often said that what you imagine is sometimes far worse than reality. That is true. Your mind can make things worse than they actually are. Because it was my mom who walked into the garage to find Jennifer, tried to get her down, and called the ambulance, she had to deal with the actual vision of that horrifying act. I only had an image in my mind based on what I had seen in movies. I had not witnessed it, but I had vivid pictures in my mind. Those images frightened me to the point where I couldn't walk into the garage any more. I wanted the door to the garage shut and locked, like something was out there which would come and get me if the door didn't remain closed.

Her bedroom, just like the garage, was another great source of fear. To get to the bathroom, I had to go past her bedroom downstairs. Mom overheard my sister and me talking one day about how we sprinted past her bedroom as fast as we could. As we ran down the stairs, we turned on every light along the way. The laundry room was right next to her bedroom. After her death I didn't go there at night, only in daylight. That's how I lived on a day-to-day basis.

Before my fear of her room became too overwhelming, I ventured in one day, deciding to prove to myself that I could go in her room to see there wasn't anything to fear. I opened the door and left it open so I could get out quickly if I had to. It was cold inside. All of her things were gone or put away, and her doll shelf was empty. The room was no longer hers, it felt empty and cold. With the closet empty and half open, I felt afraid something was waiting inside to take me, just as something had taken her. Even though the drapes were open, the room seemed dark.

I went to her mirror and looked. It was as if she was still there and I was coming to watch her curl her hair as I used to do sometimes. I wanted it to be the same. It wasn't; the good Jennifer was gone and the bad Jennifer had been left behind. There were no more dolls, her grandmother took them. Oh, how I wished there was just one doll left on the shelf, but they were all gone.

I began to feel trapped and wanted to get out, but I didn't know why. The feeling that something was going to happen to me came on all of a sudden. I ran out, shut the door, and never went back to her room again.

Not long after that, the nightmares started and I couldn't sleep.

I stayed awake just to keep the dreams away. The dreams were just like the feelings I had in her room, feelings of being trapped, empty, and cold. There was a tremendous need to run and escape in the dream as I had tried to escape Jennifer's room. They were dreams in which I fought for my life and for Jennifer's.

In the most frequent dream, I would be walking as if I were in a dark cave. Up ahead I would see Jennifer walking with her back to me and going towards a light. She was walking, but she kept stumbling and coming so close to falling that I would reach out to save her from the fall. I was always just a little too far away to save her.

I kept holding out my hand and saying, "Jennifer, come back, I will help you." But she just kept walking as if she were being pulled toward the light at the end of the tunnel or cave. The Jennifer walking was the good, vulnerable Jennifer who needed my help. As we got close to the end of the tunnel, I could see that the light we were walking towards was actually a likeness of Jennifer, but it was distorted and ugly, and it called to Jennifer and said, "Come here, come over here."

It was as if the bad image of Jennifer had some kind of control and was pulling Jennifer toward her and grabbing at her. All the while, I kept calling to Jennifer that I would help if she would wait. I called out, "No, don't go." Each night in my dreams, the good Jennifer would go to the bad one and would be taken out of my reach. I could not save her or keep her from stumbling.

The dreams became worse and worse. Each night, I would fight the bad Jennifer for the good and each night I would lose. The good Jennifer would turn around sometimes and look at me as if she wanted me to help her, but she had no control. It was like those dreams where you try to scream but nothing comes out, or you try to run but are paralyzed. I wanted to help, but I couldn't. And at the same time, I felt afraid of the bad Jennifer. There were nights I feared that, at any moment, the bad Jennifer would begin pulling me, and I would lose control.

I was afraid to tell anyone about my dreams. I didn't want to burden my mom and Bob because they were already in so much pain. I kept it to myself until I couldn't keep it in any longer.

One night my mom kept insisting I go to bed and I kept finding excuses not to. My mom didn't understand why I was being so insistent. Finally, when my mom firmly insisted, "Shari, you have to go to bed," I began to cry.

I said, "Please don't make me go in there. I can't take it one more night."

"What's the matter?"

"The nightmares, she's trying to get me, I'm afraid."

Bob and my mom tried to help me. In fact, it was Bob who

told me to imagine a floor in my mind. He said, "Take a broom and sweep that floor of all the bad images. Each time something comes into your mind that is bad, sweep it off." The sweeping helped me get to sleep, but once I was in a deep sleep, I continued to run and battle the images that frightened me.

Prior to my stepsister's death there had always been a way out of a bad situation. My mom would save me, things would change for the better, somehow I would get through. Just the fact that I made it to seventh grade proved to me that things could change. Jennifer's death showed me an irreversible side of life. This time I couldn't clean my way back to sanity or organize my room and make it all go away. I couldn't run far enough away with my dog to get away from my thoughts and fears.

Life had never been simple for me, but now the complications were suffocating. If drinking had been an option or drugs had been acceptable to me, I can see how easy it would have been to turn off my pain with something to numb my senses. Instead, I found myself using my schoolwork as my only salvation. Filling my head with science or math and the challenge it was for me to understand those things helped me to run away for awhile. The rest of the time, I stayed up late and kept myself busy with anything and everything which helped me to keep thoughts of death and fear out of my head until late at night when I had to confront them in a dream.

If we had left Bob, that house, and the whole situation, maybe things would have been different. The marriage had been in trouble for a long time. I didn't feel bold enough to tell my mom to leave, but in my heart, I wanted to.

The feeling was never so strong as one particularly difficult night. There had been a huge fight that night. In the end, we all ended up crying about Jennifer. Bob turned to me and said, "Shari, you can be my daughter now." He meant it in kindness, but my insides churned in horror. I could swear his hug would kill me, it was too tight, the reality too close. I would not be her, I would not be his daughter. I would not take her place. I didn't want to die.

I bided my time, waiting through the longest months of my life, waiting for my mom to tell us we could leave. I gave up all commitment then and detached myself from Bob, the house, and everything related. My only thoughts were of how we would escape.

That summer, we took a trip to California. I guess this trip was supposed to unify the family somehow. That trip marked the beginning of the end of my mom's and Bob's marriage.

Bob was not the same. Before Jennifer's death, living with him had its moments. Now, it was worse. His moods would swing and he was unpredictable; not unusual for a man who had just lost his child in a tragic way. But it was becoming harder and harder to live in that house, his house, any longer.

Even though we were in a car thousands of miles away from home, the tension followed us. There were arguments and disagreements over the slightest things. My mom was in the balancing act of her life. My sister and I didn't even know what she was going through until the three of us could be alone together for a short time. On one such occasion we dropped Bob and my stepbrother off, and went driving.

My mom began telling us that we needed to get out, that the marriage was over. Shawn and I encouraged her because we wanted to leave. My sister had good friends and many attachments; I, on the other hand, had absolutely nothing to leave behind. My grades were the only good thing that had happened to me while I was there, the rest was pain. I would have packed my bags then if I had the chance.

We all had different concerns about leaving, but the reality was needing to do it without anyone knowing until after we were gone. By the end of the trip we had set the date, vowing not to tell anyone except those who would help us get out. We told each other that it was just a matter of days until we would be home and could begin to collect our things.

LEAVING

It was a rainy, cloudy day when we began packing a moving van. Several friends came over after Bob went to work and we spent the rest of the day working furiously to pack our belongings before he came home. My mom spent the day crying because it meant another divorce, another mistake, another time we would have to dig up our roots and start again. We were leaving with only a few material possessions, but with experiences that would change our lives forever.

To say I was the only person thinking clearly that day would not be untrue. I was upset, but I was more concerned about getting out before Bob came home.

The roles were reversed that day, my mom became the child while I became the parent speaking reason. She was not herself and couldn't seem to make decisions. In the middle of the move, she wanted to go to a furniture store to buy a table to replace the one we would be taking. I went with her and kept saying, "Mom, what are you doing? We aren't taking anything that wasn't already ours to begin with?"

Then she would say, "But I don't want the house to seem empty." She kept repeating that. Nothing I said seemed to get through. She felt sorry for Bob, I understood that. But we had been through hell, too. We had stuck with him through the hardest times and now it was time to save ourselves.

I became frustrated with my mother. She wasn't clear on what we stood to lose. She had built our rooms with her money and supported Bob while he was out of work. She had paid for furniture, groceries, necessities, and vacations out of her earnings. We were broke, and she was going to buy him a table so he wouldn't come home to an empty space in the kitchen. I felt like an old woman telling her what to do. When my talking didn't work, I took matters into my own hands.

While my mom cried and wandered around the house, I went up into the attic of the garage and began looking through boxes for things we might need to take with us. My mom had said to forget the attic, that there was nothing up there. I went upstairs and found boxes and boxes of props and materials she used for her trade show business. Many of the materials were irreplaceable and she would need them in the future. If I had listened to her or my own fears about going into the garage, she would have walked out the door without thousands of dollars worth of business items.

I knew that once we walked out, there would be no coming back. I was right. Everything we left behind was never seen again. She left behind furniture and untold amounts of household items. We left with the bare minimum of belongings and finances. While she was feeling sorry for him, she didn't realize that maybe he wouldn't feel sorry for us when we were gone. He didn't. She made it an easy divorce and walked away without anything.

It's no wonder my sister and I took our time getting married. I could be a divorce attorney by this time, I know what you get and what you don't get. Once the tears dry up, people do whatever is necessary to stay on top.

My mom still feels the best way to handle that situation was to clear out and start again. Maybe she is right, but leaving a house filled with our belongings angered me. Maybe there wasn't much, but it belonged to us. I felt we had paid a big enough price just by living there for two years. To leave things behind was too much. That's a kid's reaction, but then again, I was just a kid.

My grandparents had a rental house that they were going to let us use, but we had to wait for the tenants to move out. All of our things were put into storage for the summer while we waited. My mom and I lived with my grandparents, while my sister stayed with friends so she could attend cheerleading practices. It had been decided that Shawn would complete the school year and continue as a cheerleader in our old district, then she would make the move to her new school in the fall; it was going to be hard for her to leave.

My mom had begun a wonderful job just months before she and Bob divorced. She was the assistant manager of what was one of the largest shopping centers in our area; she handled all the promotions and events. With my sister gone and my mom at work everyday, I found myself extremely lonely. I had my two very loving grandparents, but I felt like I was slipping into a dark cloud.

My mom and I shared a room at my grandparents' house. I found myself missing my things, wishing for some kind of security, something that would be familiar. I felt uprooted and out of control. Being able to retreat to my room with my things where I had control had been my peace and escape. Now, I couldn't do that.

The only thing still giving me comfort was my dog. I spent many afternoons washing him so he could come inside my grandma's house. When he was all sudsed up and looking like a drowned rat, I would laugh. The few laughs I had were because of Scotty.

I went inside myself that summer. I can remember the change taking place. I became even more critical of myself, even more determined to be accepted. I began to plan; every waking hour was spent planning how to get through the next year. How could I hide my past from everyone? I had decided if I kept quiet, only giving out certain pieces of information, than nobody would be able to see my differences. The feeling became very strong that I must be perfect from the moment I walked into my new school so that no one would separate me.

I began dieting. I was already thin, but to be perfect I felt I must be even thinner. Losing weight gave me a sense of control over at least one thing in my otherwise out-of-control life. If it wasn't a diet, it was making sure I had the right clothes to wear to school. If it wasn't clothes, it was my hair, skin, or constant thoughts of grades that filled my head.

Without even knowing it, I was running from the issues that were truly important. I kept my mind busy with other things so that I didn't have time to feel the deep pain. To compensate for what I saw as my faults, I was becoming a robot, trying to please everyone.

Everything I did was planned and calculated, nothing could have risk of failure or humiliation. I would stick with what I knew. I would continue to get my 4.0 because that was possible; that was the control and was acceptable. I would chastise myself for every mistake, for to be accepted, to stay alive, to make up for the past, I must be better than everyone else.

Eventually, the tenants left the rental house. It was located only twenty minutes from my mom's job and was in the middle of one of the best school districts in the state. Things were starting to come together and I looked forward to having our own place. But there was work to be done before we could move in. My mom and sister were busy, so I spent the rest of the summer with my grandparents doing odd jobs around the house and wishing I would meet someone my age. I would be weeding out in the yard and watch the kids go by on their bikes. None of them seemed to be my age, but I kept hoping.

The house was ready to move into a few days after school started and my consolation for doing work around the house was getting the biggest bedroom. Ah, to have all of my little nicknacks and treasures in their proper place, to have a place to go that was my very own.

As soon as we moved in, I began my ritual of cleaning. In fact, I sort of took over the house. I was on my own and had to be. My mom was working long hours and my sister was gone. The house became my safety zone.

I had been the one who wanted to move more than anyone else. After the first couple days of school, I started to wonder why. I knew that changing schools wouldn't be easy, but I didn't plan for it to be that hard, either. It was another place where I had to learn how to fit in and adjust.

The first day I went to school, I was wearing straight leg Levi's, a flannel shirt, Nike tennis shoes, and a velour over sweater. This outfit was a carbon copy of what everybody had been wearing at my other school. I had saved all summer and bought all the right things so that I would belong.

I received stares from the time I got on the bus in the morning to the time I got off at the end of the day. I stuck out like a sore thumb. No one wore straight legs Levis; the girls carried purses which were totally unheard of at my other school. I looked like a fish out of water.

People made it clear there wasn't a welcome wagon at this school. When I sat down in my third class of the day, the room was empty. Then two girls walked through the door. One girl was wearing flared pants and a leather jacket. She walked up to me and said, "Move."

I asked, "Why?"

She said, "I want to sit there."

I thought, "Oh, gee, yeah, that makes sense. You can't sit in my chair unless I get out of it."

else.

I thought I'd covered all the bases, I just covered them for the wrong school. Here, I had the wrong clothes, and I didn't know the slang or the rules and regulations. Those of you in junior high or high school will know what I mean when I say this. There is a way about a school, a feeling, an unwritten book that you go by to fit in. If you haven't read it, you don't belong. Nobody meant to be mean, it's just that I was new and had to earn my place.

I kept to myself from the first day on and just watched people. I knew immediately who was in and who was out. I decided I would rather be alone than be in the out group, so I just waited on the outside.

Being alone was actually the way I liked it. I would rather sit by myself than sit in the cafeteria with all the noise and commotion. Even when I had a group of friends, I found myself hating group situations. I couldn't follow the conversations because there were too many. I never knew what to say or do, and always felt that people were watching and waiting for me to make a mistake. But it wasn't them, it was me who was waiting for me to make a mistake. With me being so worried about what people thought of me and analyzing my every move, it is no wonder I preferred to be alone.

The most interesting thing is that while I kept to myself for protection, other people were making assessments about this new, quiet girl who didn't let anyone get too close. Because I never let them know any different, they thought I was a girl who walked around with life handed to her on a silver platter. They thought I was rich, that my parents bought all my clothes and that my life was easy. Sometimes not allowing people to truly know me separated me when I needed them to like me the most.

Every now and then, I wanted to shout at those who stood and made assessments. Let's see, which one do you think was a building experience: the divorces, remarriage, my stepsister's death, moving so many times, having learning disabilities? I wanted to tell them about me, and at the same time, I wanted to keep everyone from knowing I was different. I would prefer that they dislike me because I am too much than not enough.

A few months into the year, I had a couple of good friends and there was even a boy who liked me. I started to feel I fit in a little bit better. Yet it seemed that most of the girls I wanted to be friends with had been friends since they were in elementary school. Many of the girls were curious about me, and some wanted to be my friend, but they didn't want to share their friends with me.

Friendships in junior high and high school seem to be possessive and territorial, more so than any other time in your life. Some of the girls saw me as a threat to their long standing friendships, so they didn't let me into the circle. If I wanted to be friends with someone in the group, one of the girls would say, "Well, I was friends with her first." Fortunately, a couple of people didn't care whether their territory was being invaded or fear that a new person would mean fewer friends for them. In fact, the one or two friends

I had, were true friends; I still have them to this day.

Growing up and being in junior high is like having the biggest hormone change of your life, everything is such a big deal. I came home crying so many times saying, "Mom, why don't I have any friends, why don't I fit in?" While I was doing that, I bet the people who wouldn't let me into their group were saying the same thing to their mothers. It is a part of life, searching for a place to belong. It's just that in my case, my need to fit in was amplified by the years of truly not fitting in at all.

CHAPTER
13

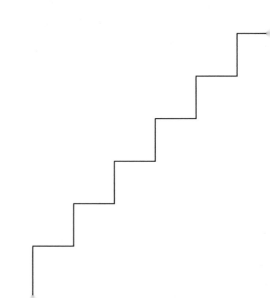

SICKNESS AND HEALTH

By the end of October, my sister made plans to move into our house. When she came home, it was strange. I was beginning a new life and beginning to be settled, and now she was being uprooted. I tried to relate with what she was feeling but I couldn't. My outlook on life was improving in this new place.

I had waited for Shawn to come home, looking forward to having a companion. Instead, we hardly ever talked. I guess I had also become used to living alone. It had been peaceful even though it was lonely. When Shawn came home and was unhappy, it wasn't what I had expected, and I was sad that my dream of a little happy home with just the three of us was not turning out like I thought it would.

The stress of the move was obvious in all of us, but especially my sister and my mom. By the time the new school year began, my mom was diagnosed with diverticulitis and colitis, two serious intestinal diseases. Having one is bad enough, having both of them means that they work against each other making it impossible to eat even the most common foods without having an attack of severe pain. I watched my mom go from eating regular food to eating baby food in a matter of months. She was in constant pain and was never without her medication.

I'm sure there are many causes for these diseases, but for my mom I know it was stress. The pain that she didn't show on the outside went inward and tore her apart.

Watching my mom double up in pain over the steering wheel on the way out of the garage was a very frightening experience. I had visions of the future without her whenever this happened. What would I do, where would I go? Losing one person made me see the possibility and the reality of losing another.

When I was older, she told me how frightened she was during this time. She was more worried about what would happen to us if she died than what would happen to her. She was a woman alone again, raising us by herself, but more than that she was a woman with learning disabilities. That was the key element. So much of the reason for her insecurity was that she could create a production and make it happen better than anyone else; she just couldn't fill out an insurance form.

Here was an intelligent woman, a creative, beautiful woman, who was seriously ill, raising two daughters on her own and starting over again for the third time. She must have wondered how it got this way. She told me several years ago that at one point during that year, she ended up in the hospital during the middle of one of her shows. She was so ill she thought sure she was going to die, the difference was that she didn't care anymore. She had lost the fight to live. She woke up the next morning in the hospital - she had lived despite herself.

She never told me of this incident until I was older but somehow, I knew. All you had to do was look in her eyes, she wasn't the same person anymore. She didn't have the same energy or life that she had even a year before. Without ever telling her, I feared losing her every moment I was awake.

I became obsessed with her health. She could not eat solid foods for almost a year and I watched her like a hawk. I monitored every bit of food that entered her mouth, not only for her, but also for myself. I became the health food and vitamin expert, even going so far as to eat what she ate. Although I ate some solid food, I, too, would eat yogurt and baby food.

I don't know why I did it. I was in eighth grade and should have been eating twinkies and dingdongs; instead, I was shopping at nutrition centers. I think I did it because I needed to be involved with my mom's recovery. If I had stood on the outside watching her pain, it would have killed me. Being involved made me feel more in control than standing by and watching the illness happen.

She became extremely thin during that first year in our new home. My mom had a weight problem up to that point so everyone said, "You look so good." I thought she looked good, but not happy. She cared when she started to pick up weight again, but I didn't. I only cared that the life came back into her eyes when the pain started to go away and she could eat normal food again.

When you look at all the pictures from that year, we all had eyes that were drawn and spiritless. We smiled but you could still sense something was wrong.

My sister had been in her new school for only four days when she was nominated for homecoming princess. She was only in the school five days when she was asked to homecoming. She was in school for only three weeks when she became ill with mononucleosis. High levels of stress made her weak with exhaustion; she was out of school more than she had been in because of the illness.

The pain goes somewhere; Shawn had given up a lot. Friends, school, cheerleading. Then she moved into a new house and a new school and had work to catch up on. The stress must have been incredible. In all that we had gone through I had hardly ever heard Shawn discuss how she really felt about any of it, especially my stepsister's death. She took it in and handled it but the pain had to be inside there somewhere hurting her.

Shawn eventually went back to school and I was beginning to consider myself the healthiest of the bunch. But when you look at pictures from that Christmas and compare them to those from a year earlier, you can see the telltale signs. Without my knowing it, I had mononucleosis. My glands were swollen out like a bull frog. I thought my face was just gaining weight. Now, when I look at the pictures, I think I must have been blind not to see the size of my neck and not know something was wrong.

In my case, the virus just stayed in my system and grew worse without manifesting itself as an illness until March or April of that year. My illness was also stress related, similar to my mother's problems. I plowed through my school work making A's in every class through two trimesters. I studied every night with flashcards and a tape recorder.

I was little Miss Perfect, handing in assignments at the right time, working ahead in the book, raising my hand in class. I became known as the smart kid. Nobody went home with me at night, so they didn't know what I had to do to get the A's. I kept to myself and people only knew my grade if they asked me, but I took pride in being able to say I got an A. It was more than pride, it was everything to me. I threw myself into my work to keep from thinking of my mom's illness or anything else for that matter. It was a way for me to control something, when everything else was out of my control.

As much as my grades meant to me, I began to feel that something was missing. I would look at myself and believe that I was never good enough, and this feeling would cloud each goal and each step I took. I belittled and criticized myself after every award, and replayed every mistake over and over again. It became compulsive self-criticism as time went on. I was so hard on myself that just living was impossible because nothing I did was ever right.

I did everything thinking that when I crossed that next line things were going to get better for me, as if an award or an "A" could erase my pain. Sometimes life did get better but I was so caught up in low self-esteem that I didn't even see the change. I was obsessed with the next step that would bring me acceptance.

HAMSTER ON A WHEEL

After I figured out the amount of time and effort I had to put in on a daily basis to keep my grades, I decided that wasn't enough. I had the system of studying down and could handle it. I wanted more. I wanted to become a cheerleader. I thought cheerleaders were happy all the time, with no problems and instant popularity. The grass was greener where the cheerleaders stood.

I feel as though I should have said, "And now for my next trick...." The fact that I had achieved high grades was sort of a balancing act and now I was going to try for something which would require me to do the things I feared most. Risk failure, use my motor skills, and be coordinated all at once? Who me?

I chose cheerleading because it was something I was familiar with. I had watched my sister for years. I watched her skill as a cheerleader, but I think I was more interested in what I thought being a cheerleader brought to you. Shawn always had friends and was always going somewhere exciting. For years I lived vicariously through her awards, achievements, and excitement. I think I had thought grades would bring that same excitement into my life. It brought respect, but not excitement. I was not disappointed with my success in school, I just came to want more for myself.

As the tryouts grew closer, I still maintained that I would try out. But a fear welled up inside of me that was amazing. With each passing day, I realized I might fail. Before, when I had little or no success in school, I didn't have anything to lose by trying. Now that I had established myself as successful in a particular area, it became safe, I had control over it. I had no guarantees with cheerleading. No control whatsoever. With the possibility of failure looming over my head, I wondered if I should try out at all.

It was quite a dilemma. Play it safe and not get what I want or try to get what I want and risk the possibility of failure. I put so much pressure on myself it is not hard to understand why my body gave way to full-blown mononucleosis just a few days before cheer tryouts started.

My sister, Mom, and I went on a week long trip to California during our spring break from school. During the trip, I practiced cheers at each stop along the way, knowing I would have to be prepared by the first day back in school. Each night I would worry and worry about whether or not I would make it, and every day I would practice more cheers.

I found myself extremely tired. By Thursday of that week, I had a horrible sore throat and had to lie down after the slightest bit of exertion. By Friday, I was on a plane home to my father's apartment until my mom and sister could drive home to get me.

I became ill and had to be hospitalized for most of the following week. I lost weight rapidly, I was achy, and tired to the point of exhaustion after only small movements. Even while in the hospital with an IV hanging out of my arm, I had my mom contact the school to assure them that I would be back in time to try out for cheerleading. Even with this amount of illness I was still driven.

I lay in the hospital crying, knowing I probably wouldn't make it back to school in time to try out. I cried because it would be two years until I had a chance at the high school to try out again. I imagined myself getting through the next two years being unpopular because I wasn't a cheerleader. Do you see the distortion? I was sure that if I wasn't a cheerleader, nobody would like me.

208

Had I tried out and not made it, I would have been hard on myself for failing; now I was angry and frustrated at myself for becoming ill.

My learning disabilities made me doubt myself. I was sure if something went wrong it was because of my not seeing it, hearing it, or being aware of it. No report card changed that feeling. Cheerleading couldn't change it. You would have to go back to my childhood and change the very experiences that molded these thoughts; an absent father, failures in school, inconsistencies in my education and few if any answers or help for my learning problems. Then add the death of my stepsister, the subsequent divorce and my mother's recent illness and you have a child who is sure if she was just a little bit more, everything would be great. Coming in now and saying, "Shari, don't be so hard on yourself," was too late.

My mom tried to tell me to slow down. A lot of people tried to tell me to slow down, but I didn't listen. My mom actually consulted a medical doctor once and asked him to tell me to stop pushing myself so hard in school and related activities.

The doctor knew that my heavy work load at school was the likely cause of my chronic stomach problems and other stress related problems. But he found it hard to say, "Stop getting good grades, Shari." I don't blame him. If it had been drugs or an eating disorder, it would have made his job much easier. Instead, all he could do was tell me to stop studying so hard. What the doctor didn't know was that I was relentless with myself. It seemed a simple problem from the outside, but it was a whole variety of problems that tore my insides apart with worry.

After I left the hospital, I spent a month at home recovering. Teachers were good enough to send my work home to me by way of friends. The rest at home was both a blessing and a curse. When I was really sick, I couldn't even think about anything, so I got some rest and even enjoyed the peace. I didn't have to compete and didn't even feel well enough to worry. As I started to feel better, I woke up. Life was going on. I began to worry that when I went back to school, people would have forgotten the new girl. I would not be a cheerleader, and I had been sick for a month. Once again, I was managing to find something to be concerned about.

This new worry of disappearing into obscurity made me push myself to go back to school before I was physically ready. I was pale, trembling, and extremely thin, but I went back. I went back with a speech in my hand and banners to place around the school. I couldn't become a cheerleader but I had asked one of my teachers when the campaigns for school president started and began preparing everything for that date. I went back on the day the introductory speeches were made. I probably should have stayed home another week, but I was bound and determined, obsessed with needing to be more. If I wasn't one thing, then I would be another.

I didn't win or even make it into the finals. You see, people usually vote for the people they know. I was new that year plus I had been out of school for a month. Nobody knew me. Now I think back and wonder why being less than the top wasn't good enough for me? Why didn't I just run for treasurer, why president?

I went from that race to another. The next available position was Pep Club President. Not a big deal, but I thought if I was elected, I could make it into something.

There were only two people running, six people voting and it was a tie. Talk about knocking your self-esteem for a loop. With only six people voting, I still couldn't get elected. The advisor of the Pep Club made an executive decision and made me and the other girl that ran, co-presidents. I was crushed. I guess I was thankful she didn't call a re-vote. I wondered what the chances were that I would have lost.

That year, I missed cheer tryouts, ran for president of the school and lost, tried out for the track team and dropped out when I realized that I might lose a race now and then, and then ran for Pep Club President managing to tie with only six voters. I even read for a school play, but I sat in the back of the room in an obscure spot, afraid that if I was called on, I might stumble over a word. When the drama coach finally found me, he had me read one line, I didn't make the cast and then wondered why.

Look at the pattern. I searched for my identity through a cheer sweater or a title after my name. I don't even know if I wanted to be president, I just wanted to be liked. I didn't even have the skills to be a cheerleader at the time. I was scared out of my mind to face a panel of judges and the possibility of failure, but I was willing to go to any extreme to find recognition and praise. I went into everything looking for my value and ended up feeling like less than before.

At the same time I was learning to sabotage myself with worry, fear, illness, and stress. Getting sick and worrying all the time helped to keep me from doing anything which might result in a large failure. It also kept me from any chance of success. I didn't consciously say, "That's it, I am going to wreck my chances," it just sort of happened. I was afraid, so I made my world very small by refusing to take risks. If I was sick or somehow incapacitated, I thought I hadn't failed, I just didn't try. But not trying or sabotaging myself with the fear of failure, was my real failure.

That's the trouble with worry and fear. We will all fail. I see in my life now, that it was my mistakes that taught me the most and made me strong. When you live with guilt, worry, and fear, there is a tendency to hide from the world and its ability to overwhelm you. Everybody does it, but it is particularly easy for a learning disabled person to hide behind these emotions. To say that we can't or that we don't want to, or that the world is against us, excludes us from trying. The excuses are useless. "My teacher in fifth grade called me stupid." "I can't read very well." "My father was an alcoholic." We could go on forever lamenting our situation, or we can try to get out of it.

I ran away from the chance of success as much as I ran away from failure. I was learning that as much as people dislike a loser, they also don't seem to like people who are too successful. I made my world very small and protected, but completely miserable. No success was good enough, every failure was the end of the world. Living is not an easy proposition, but it is easier if you go for what you want in life rather than sitting around wondering about what you could have been if you had just seized the moment, stopped the excuses, and did something about your situation. So easy to say now.

JUST ONE PERSON

That year I spent a lot of time in my Language Arts/Social Studies teacher's room. Her door was open at lunch time so I just started going in one day. Even when I had friends to sit with at lunch, I found it much more peaceful to sit in a quiet room, read a book, or talk to one person rather than be overwhelmed by so many voices in the cafeteria.

Without questions or comment she let me come in and sit with her. We would even eat lunch together sometimes. Other times, we would just not say anything at all while eating. This was a woman who could have said, "Sorry, I just have too much to do to have anyone come into my room during lunch." It would have been her perogative, it was her preparation period. Instead, I found a friend in her. I didn't tell her my life story, she didn't tell me her's, we were just quiet friends at a time when I was lonely.

When kids my age would laugh at a joke or a story, I somehow felt removed. I didn't find the same things funny anymore. I didn't feel that I fit in with people my own age. Being around adults allowed me to be myself. With the right adult I didn't have to feel "on" or have to entertain anyone. I could be quiet and not have to work so hard. Somehow, I looked at adults and thought, "If you could read my mind, I think you would truly understand." I could not say that about my peers.

It was my Social Studies/Language Arts teacher who gave me one of the most important gifts of that year. When she told me that she had recommended me for a new English and Social Studies honors program, it was like being validated. For the first time in my life, I was being picked out as having exceptional abilities. You couldn't pay enough for the feeling it gave me. A teacher, someone who I respected so much, believing in me so strongly. Other kids invited into the program took it in stride; to me, it was the reason for all the late nights studying. I was finally being recognized as being smart rather than just a hard worker.

My mom was concerned about the extra work load. I was, too; being in an honors class meant you had twice the assignments. I thought about it and, to me, the amount of time I spent doing more homework would be worth the word "honors" after my grade on my report card.

Students in those two classes were set apart. Even though people might make a joke when we left the regular classroom to go to honors classes with remarks like, "there go the egg-heads," there was respect in there somewhere. Maybe it was just me. I respected myself for the first time and that was more important than what other people thought.

ON MY OWN

There were a few trials with teachers that year. When things went wrong, I was lucky to have a counselor, or I could always confide in my Language Arts/Social Studies teacher. But there were also times when I just had to handle life on my own.

I started math at the beginning of the year, carrying over the great success that I had in seventh grade. I was hoping I would be lucky and have another good teacher. Even though I could learn fairly well in my new math class, I found myself intimidated by my new teacher. Her teaching style was good, but at the same time, her personality was often very gruff. Other times she was flamboyant and outspoken. I didn't know exactly how to react to her. I spent a lot of time being scared in her class simply because I didn't know what to expect.

Without meaning any harm, she sometimes would make examples of people in class. I often needed extra help or wanted to ask questions in class, but was afraid to because I didn't want to be singled out.

I struggled on in silence until finally I ended up crying every night at the kitchen table trying to figure out my math by myself. I finally decided to wait until after class to explain to the teacher that I needed more help.

The next day, I waited until the rest of the class was gone and I approached the teacher's desk. I was nervously shuffling my feet when she raised her head to ask what I wanted. I said, "Well, I have this problem called dyslexia, so it takes me longer to learn.

It's because of my dyslexia that I tend to ask more questions and need more help than most of the other kids."

Then I waited for her response which wasn't what I expected. She became loud and said, "Don't give me that excuse!"

I thought, "Uh-oh, here it comes."

"You aren't going to use that excuse in this room with me. Don't use dyslexia as a crutch."

I started to approach it from a different angle but her mind was set. I would start to say something, but she would shake her head. I was getting A's in her class. I wondered what would happen to a person who was getting C's and tried to explain.

I came home crying and explained the whole situation to my mom. This was not a new occurrence; I shouldn't have been shocked. And yet, being misunderstood, even the thought of someone saying I was using my learning problems as an excuse, made me angry and hurt. If I was using my learning problems as an excuse, then why was I getting A's in the class, why was I turning in all of my homework?

When people tell you something like that, you want to shout at them that they have no idea what they are saying. You want to tell them that unless they walk around for a day with you, that they don't know what it is like. They don't know what it is like to face a teacher and try to explain a problem that the teacher doesn't believe exists. Only to have that teacher - a person you look up to - slap you in the face with words like "crutch," "excuse," or "lazy." My mom took the next step and had a conference with this teacher. She explained the whole thing and asked if the teacher would be willing to give me an extra minute or two so I could absorb the information. In the end, she made an effort with me in class; I ended up respecting her and she understood my learning problems.

Don't give up out there. You may have had similar experiences. Talk about it before you give up. The teacher couldn't read my mind. I looked perfectly normal, so she thought I wasn't trying. We got off on the wrong foot but that didn't mean it had to stay that way. If you're having trouble with teachers, talk to them.

THE JOURNAL

You would have to get inside of a child's head to know what makes her feel good or bad. As much as I loved my teachers that year, there was one particular event which made me ask, "How would you feel if you were me?" To most, the incident will go unremembered, but to me it is a great lesson about the differences in what people value.

As I said earlier, I was a collector of things, like dolls, old clothes, toys, books, and school papers. I don't know what I thought would happen if I threw something away, but I still continued to be a saver. As we moved and our lives changed, I couldn't let go of cards, gifts, and personal items; they were like a little piece of me and my loved ones. What if I lost that person and didn't have the letter or the gift to hold onto? I kept everything.

It was new for me to keep school papers. In elementary school I usually just kept the items I liked the best. By junior high, I was keeping everything. It was my work, and to throw it away was like throwing all of my efforts away. I kept a box, an overflowing box of papers, which chronicled my years in school. They were a part of me, a piece of my life was spent doing that particular paper or project. Someone else could do a paper in a short time and not invest as much into it; I put my blood, sweat, and tears into it and I wanted to keep it. It was worth that much to me.

During my eighth grade year, we were asked to do a project on the Westward Movement. We were to write a journal of the long and often fatal journey of wagon trains taking people to a new life in the West. To teach us about their lives and hardships and how it related to populating the Western United States, we were asked to write a story to report the facts of the movement in fictional form. The book itself was to look like it could have been found in the wagon train. The pages were to be aged in some way and we were to do anything and everything to make the book look and sound authentic.

We were given two months to do the project which meant that we had to organize our time to get it done by the due date. In eighth grade, it was considered the biggest and hardest project we would do the whole year, and it was something we all looked upon with some fear and dread.

Once the project was started, it actually was fun and a great learning experience. With expectations ranging from thirteen to one hundred pages, you literally could do the report the night before, but you couldn't do the job that could get you an A.

I can't remember a project I worked harder on or enjoyed more. I spent the first part of the month and a half actually writing the journal of a young girl on the Westward trail. She was the storyteller sharing her family's perils through her letters back home as well as through her diary. When I first came home I said, "Mom, how am I going to write this? How can I be a storyteller?"

She said, "Why don't you just be you? Be a little girl making a journey with her family. The diary can be a collection of letters to her family and friends back home." Now there was something I could relate to. After all, I had just left my home and my school and was living in a different place than I had the year before. I knew what it was like to move and leave behind people I really cared about. I became the little girl in my story.

My first letter of the journal was to say good-bye to all of my family and friends as we set out on a long and unsure journey. I said the same words in the letter that I had said to my friends when I said good-bye in fifth grade.

When I first brought the assignment home and described it to my mom, I showed her the list of events that had to appear in my story. I could pick from a list of about forty events and I had to include twenty or more in my project. There were some things that had to be included; the death of a loved one on the trail, and meeting people of different backgrounds and religions to signify the melting pot of people looking for a new home. The rest of the story could be made up with the help of a history book.

When my mom looked at the list, she was quick to notice that there were some things that would be very painful to write about. For instance, if someone from our family had to die on the trail, who would it be? I certainly wouldn't want to write about a sister dying, and I couldn't even think of losing my mother.

My mom was relieved to see that I had chosen to lose a friend that I had met on the trail. I wrote about how my friend had died and how we were forced to bury him on the trail and leave him behind. In the story, I made a cross of sticks and branches to use as a headstone for his grave. I wrote of the emotion of being pulled away from the gravesite, crying because I didn't want to leave him. My mom can remember reading what I had written about my friend dying out on the trail and realizing it was actually my way of relating the pain from the loss of my stepsister.

In each circumstance and through each story, I was blending in my own personal feelings and emotions. My mother in the story was much like my own mother in real life. I had an image from which to draw her character. My mom in the story was even sick on the journey, which also had a touch of reality in it.

When it came to deciding on the type of person that my fictional father should be, I decided on a minister. I think I chose a minister because then the parents would be less likely to get a divorce. A minister meant a family man, a strong father figure, and in some way it signified safety and stability in my character's home life, which was exactly what I was looking for in my own life.

To make the journal look authentic, I took blank, white sheets of paper and dipped them in tea. I then put them on cookie sheets to dry in a warm oven. When the paper dried, I turned a burner on low and slowly turned the paper up against the burner until all the edges had been burned. I filled the kitchen with smoke on a couple of occasions but the papers looked authentic.

After I had copied my story onto the tea stained pages, my mom helped me make a quilted cover for the outside. It was made of a calico type material, the kind Melissa Gilbert wore on "Little House On The Prairie." We put boards inside the fabric, tied ribbon on the side for a binding and covered the edges in tea soaked lace. When we were done, it definitely looked like a little girl's diary and definitely was aged to the point that it could have been on a wagon moving westward early in our history.

I carried my Westward Movement journal to school wrapped in plastic like it was a king's ransom. I had spent a lot of time on the project, researching it, writing it, and finally creating the look of the diary itself.

I turned in my project amid the groans of those who had stayed up all night working on their journals. We were all relieved to finish it and most were looking forward to getting our grades and our journals back.

About a month and a half later we got our grades, but no journals were returned. We were told they were being kept so that people wouldn't copy them the next year. I protested and so did others; we had spent so many hours, literally months of work and we wanted them back. The teachers who assigned this project to their students told us they might change their minds by the end of the year and we should check back. Months passed, and I kept asking until my teacher finally said she had thrown them away, and if they hadn't all been thrown away she didn't know where they were.

I was so mad I asked if I could go through the storage closet to see if they might have stored some there. She let me go through all the boxes but there were no Westward Journals to be found. I was heartbroken. To them, it was just another Westward Movement journal; to me, it was the only one I had ever done.

To say I was angry is quite an understatement, but my mom was even angrier. She had watched the work and time spent preparing that project. Just as parents keep finger paintings and pictures brought home from school, my mom took pride in my work and my accomplishments. She wanted the journal and the story I had written as much as I did.

I can remember one day my mom drove me to school and asked when I would be getting my report back. When I told her they had thrown them away, she was going to march in and speak to my teacher. I stopped her. "It's no use, they threw them away long ago. Mom, I like my teacher, I don't want to start something. Let's just let it go and from now on, I'll ask ahead of time what the teacher is going to do with our papers after they have been graded." The problem is I never did another project like that, I have nothing to equal it. I will never forget those words, "I threw it away!"

Remember this story. If you are a parent, take note of your child's work when they bring it to you, or there will come a time when they won't bring it to you anymore. If you're a teacher, remember it may be your zillionth report, but it is the only one from that student. If you throw it away or treat it like it's nothing, why should your students work so hard to meet your requirements? Things like this happen in classrooms everyday. There are wonderful teachers, thinking of great assignments that don't just teach students how to memorize or spit out what they have been told in true or false answers. The assignments force you to think about what you are learning. You spend months of your time putting together something you are proud of, putting pieces of yourself into the project. If your work is thrown away, all the good that was built into the assignment has just been ruined.

Just as red ink emphasizes that you have made a mistake, continued red ink becomes all you start to see. Just as assignments are given to teach a certain subject, throwing a project in the garbage takes away the meaning of the assignment and the value of the work. Just as children are taught to respect the rights and property of others, to trust adults, to take pride in their work and to achieve, throwing away their work just to prevent the possibility of someone else cheating, sends a mixed signal about what you expect from them.

In some way, make the ink a different color, the marks on the paper a little lighter. Show me I made a mistake, but also, please show me with pretty colors what I did right. Display my work and show me that it is valuable rather than throwing it away, that even in its early stages any skill is worth building on.

THE LAST DAY OF SCHOOL

The end of school had come and once again I was feeling the waves of relief coming over me. Another year down; another nine months checked off the calendar.

The 4.0 remained intact and I was exhausted from the struggle. I was ready to enjoy a summer with the friends I had made that year. All I could think of on the bus ride to school the last day was summer days without my books.

There had been only a few crises that year. My mom was alive, doing well, and her job was keeping her busy. My sister had adjusted to her school and had made the varsity cheer squad for the upcoming year. The problems we had seemed small compared to a year before. Now that a little time had passed even a lost cheer squad position or bid for school president didn't seem so bad. My biggest problem at the time was something I didn't even realize or fully understand.

In my hurry to get through the year and recover from my illness, I had again missed some subtle hints of change along the way. While I was sick and then recovering, even when I had come back to school and was muddling my way back through the ranks of junior high, I didn't realize that the boundaries of friendships had changed since I was gone. Although I thought people would be glad to have me back and I was looking forward to seeing them, life had moved ahead while I was gone.

Instead of coming back to school and re-cultivating my friends, I had one goal and one goal only, to *"be somebody."* And if that meant running for president of my school or running off a cliff, I probably would have done it.

On the last day of school, I noticed that I was sitting alone at the annual-signing party in the gymnasium. Again, at a table full of girls and boys at an ice cream parlor after school that day, I sat virtually alone in a room full of people. Nobody talked to me. I thought, "They must hate me." I blew it up to be bigger than life. In actuality, no one really knew me. I was a girl who was driven, a girl who measured herself by the awards after her name. In the process I didn't let anyone get near me. Some were jealous because they thought I had it all. Most just didn't understand me. I didn't even understand me.

That day I went home from school and cried wondering, "Why doesn't anyone like me?" Being shunned even if only slightly became my crisis for the day.

Whether I knew it or not, crisis was my cycle. Once you have lived with crisis and turmoil, you feel something is wrong when it isn't there. It's almost as if it is a way to live; worry and crisis were what I knew best. Feeling rejected and cast aside were what I knew. If rejection or crisis wasn't there, I created it. Children of divorce, of alcoholics, or children with learning disabilities - anyone who has lived with crises - know what I am talking about. The crisis, the pain, as much as you want to live without it, no one has taught you how. Maybe you feel it might not be possible to live without pain, maybe you think that everyone lives like this. I didn't think others lived this way, I just didn't think I could live any other way.

With that feeling in mind, I created my own escape from the world. I would escape the real worlds harsh judgements of me, which were really my own. I would escape the world where I didn't seem to fit and where bad things happened. I would go into my own single focus of pushing, shoving and perfection only to come out and find that nothing had really changed. The isolation of my room, the teacher's room at school, the plaque on the wall, the cheer sweater, my need for success, these were my escapes and at times, isolated me from the very people who could have been my friends and isolated me from people at a time when I really needed them.

I didn't realize then that I had the power to make my life the way I wanted it to be, right in the palm of my hand. The fragile child I was didn't realize that crisis wasn't always necessary.

Actually, that summer was not as bad as I expected. I mended some friendships and spent some time at our cabin. Most importantly, a man came into my mother's life who would also have a great effect on mine. Through him, I became aware, if only in part, of the kind of personal strength that lay inside me.

CHAPTER 14

Jack, my mother's new boyfriend, was a highly successful business man and restauranteur. He had great stories and a great sense of humor, but more than that, he was extremely kind and gentle.

At this point in my life, I was skeptical of anyone who entered our lives. I lost my trust in people. I was sure that what had happened before could happen again if we were not careful. But Jack was different. He did not smother me with kindness, nor did he make me feel fearful. He was a friend to my mother and a friend to me. I watched him nurse my mom back to health. Although I entered into any relationship with him cautiously at first, over time I realized that this man was genuine.

Because of his restaurant background he was very knowledgeable about the health foods, vitamins, and minerals that my mom needed to recover from her intestinal problems. What he didn't know, he researched; and he bought books for her to read. He bought juicers and powdered foods, and a variety of vitamins filled the cupboards of our small kitchen. It seemed his primary goal was to restore her health.

When she first met him, my mom was very thin. Her eyes were growing lifeless, and she clung to her medicine bottles as though they were life itself. She existed on baby food and liquids. Within months of his help, she started to recover. The doctors had done the underlying work, but he knew that the real cure involved a new lifestyle and a whole new diet to fully restore her health.

Because he was my mom's boyfriend, I probably should have been distant. Instead, I spent a lot of time with the two of them watching and learning. By the time their relationship ended, my mom was eating solid food again and had life in her eyes. Had that been all it would have been plenty, but in addition to healing the body he also taught my mom and I some valuable lessons about life.

For me the real message from him was about what he called "Positive Motivation." They were the buzz words of the time, with books, tapes, and positive motivational speakers around every corner. Although there are still motivational speakers, books and tapes, it seemed everyone came out of the woodwork in the late seventies and early eighties with ideas on how people could change their lives by changing their attitudes. Jack had heard all the latest, but what he gave me were a few basic ideas that would change my way of thinking drastically.

I began to think of my mind as a tape recorder. At that point in my life, the "tape" I played was filled with pain because I was sad, self-critical, and had a negative view of myself. I often felt as though I would collapse under the weight of my own criticism. But the message Jack brought to me was that my tape didn't have

221

to play the same old negative information. I could actually reprogram what I was saying to myself and start a whole new "self-talk."

I learned that it really doesn't take much to reprogram your tape recorder. All you have to do is want to change. I didn't have to buy an expensive program or read a lot of books to learn how to say better things to myself or set goals for my future. All I did was listen to Jack tell me a few simple tips. Then I began putting those things to use that very summer.

My life didn't change immediately, but over time subtle changes became life changes and have remained part of my way of keeping on track.

CHANGING THE TAPE RECORDING

As a very small child, I often heard the phrase "Love your neighbor as yourself." What I failed to realize is that you can't love and care for others until you love and care about yourself. The way you see others and the way they view you is all based on how you feel about you! If your tape recorder is loaded with a negative self image and a belief that you are incapable of achieving the goals you have set for yourself, you have a foolproof prescription for failure. The only way to change the outcome is to change the tape!

I found myself caught up in brutal self-talk, filled with worry and fear of everything from rejection to failure. I lived each day thinking that if something bad hadn't happened, sooner or later that would change. It was a kind of "Murphy's Law" way of living; everything that can go wrong eventually will go wrong. Even though I was succeeding in school, I convinced myself that the only way to continue to be successful was to be extremely hard on myself.

There is a difference between pushing yourself to be the best you can be and pushing yourself with guilt, shame, and fear of failure. I was successful but did not laugh; I was achieving but did not enjoy my achievements. I was so filled with pain and fear of failure that each stride forward was coupled with a step back.

I knew that self-criticism wasn't right, and I felt terrible day in and day out because I could never let up on myself. I knew I wanted to change, but had become so used to the focus on failure that I thought it was the only way to live. I didn't feel I deserved to talk "positively" to myself. Whenever I started to feel too good or have a little bit of fun, I would start thinking about a test that I had to study for, a paper that still wasn't finished, my relationship with my dad, or any number of things which would bring me back to my cycle of worry and fear.

Jack told me, "If you think negative, then negative things will happen. If you believe you won't ever be anything and concentrate your efforts on being a failure, you probably won't make it." It's called a self-fulfilling prophecy. You say it will happen or someone else tells you it will happen, and somehow it does. It's as if without wanting to, you set yourself up for failure.

I did it every day. I was so hard on myself, it's amazing that I did succeed. If I had gone easier on myself, I could have enjoyed life more and even made room for other things I enjoyed doing. Instead, I made my world very small. I would only do challenging things if I felt I had nothing to lose. I always left myself an "out." I prepared myself for failure because I was sure I would fail.

Jack told me to change what I was telling myself, literally to reprogram the tape recording in my head with positive messages. At first I thought that this idea is so silly, so simple. Then I thought if it is so simple, why am I not doing it?

THINKING POSITIVE

The more positive your outlook, the more likely it is that good things will happen. When you are sure something can't happen, how likely is it you will try out every possibility, work every angle, and see a project through? Saying something can't be done is an easy way out. I'm sure every recording artist, rock star, actor, writer, and business person thought many times that success was impossible. If they thought it was impossible long enough, they never would have made it; but at some point they just said, "Maybe there is another way I haven't tried, another door I haven't knocked on."

Jack had become successful by filling the gaps in the restaurant world. To all the people who said it was impossible, he closed his ears. He made it, and he told me about many others who succeeded because they refused to stay down. Their setbacks only inspired them to try harder, until they achieved their goals.

Jack's words would have meant nothing if he didn't also live them. With him nothing was impossible. He was good to my mother and was convinced she was going to get well. Instead of watching her be sick, he started taking action.

He lived with hope and optimism. He didn't let the problems of life get to him as I had seen other people do. Everyone has problems, but he seemed to be steady all the time, none of the extreme highs and lows that I had experienced. He glided through life and always seemed happy and easy going. I wanted to know how. How do you become successful in business? How do you stay happy? Why are you optimistic all the time?

My mom would not date someone who didn't include my sister and I in their relationship. My sister wasn't around all that much so it was usually me who needed to be included. Without reservation he not only included me, but became one of the first gentle and caring male figures in my life. He was easy to trust and cared deeply. He made me laugh, but most of all he talked to me. That was so important. He talked to me about changes he had made in his life, how he changed the way he thought about himself, and how I could do the same.

Maybe he did this without realizing the kind of impact he had on me, but it was a very important time in my life. I was searching and wanted to change. He could have been just another man but he was different; he let me get near him. He started to plant the idea that maybe some men were trustworthy and I could actually form an attachment with them. It was just a spark, but I needed it.

He lived the lessons he taught me and explained how to change the negative patterns in my head into positive selftalk. I had to learn how to override the negative talk with positive talk.

For example, I tended to go around saying to myself things like, "Don't trip," "Don't say something dumb," "Don't fail," "You don't look good enough today." In the midst of all those awful words there was no room for any positives. Jack said I should think of some positive statements (now I also use Bible verses) to replace the negative phrases I was saying to myself. In time you get so used to saying the positive over and over to yourself, it becomes a habit just like the negative did.

I started saying, "You look great today! I feel good about myself! I am an excellent student!" over and over again. At first I thought, "That's conceited, silly, and even dumb!" I had every reason not to do it, but I figured I didn't have anything to lose. I kept repeating it to myself and eventually it worked. It felt a lot better than saying, "You look awful today, you are ugly, you are stupid."

I decided that when school started again I was going to change my attitude about school, too. Now if at the same time I didn't also apply myself and study hard, all the positive statements in the world would not make a difference. The point here is that positive self-talk alone will not solve all your problems. You have to do the studying and preparations, but positive self-talk will give you the right attitude that will help lead to success.

My problem was that even when I studied hard, I would go into the test or quiz with such a feeling of panic and fear of failure that it made it hard for me to concentrate. If I could replace that with a feeling of confidence, I could save myself a lot of extra credit work to make up for low test scores!

You set yourself up for what you want. Tell yourself what you want to be and that's what you will become. From the first day I tried using positive self-talk, I could see the difference. The day was a little easier to get through. I wasn't as exhausted or fatigued as I had been before. School would be the ultimate test, but for now summer was giving me good practice for the year ahead.

I must say that the negative habits I had were hard to break at first. If I stopped the positive thoughts, there were floods of negatives ready to come in. Be prepared for that to happen. In time it will get easier, when you learn to counteract that old voice with a whole new one.

Changing the tape recording was really only a surface remedy. The things I'm telling you in this section are not cure-alls. Counseling was my true relief; I had to dig deep to get rid of my pain. To make a change, you have to start somewhere. Maybe you don't have a lot of deep dark stuff hidden somewhere to be dealt with; maybe you have just become used to sabotaging yourself and living with a bad self-image. Whatever your situation, just start somewhere. That's what I did. Any positive step you take will be awkward, even scary, but it will pay off with time.

When you are trying to change the way you feel about yourself, there is not just one "right" way to do it. You may find it necessary to write some of your positive statements down to really make them stick. As a learning disabled person, I have found that writing things down either in list form or in a journal has been extremely helpful. Let go of what other people might think, the old habits, the comfort in failure, and see what you could be if you really believed that anything was possible.

SETTING GOALS

Another valuable lesson I learned from Jack was the importance of goal setting. By setting and achieving goals you can see yourself progress and improve in a tangible way. If I really thought about it, I could say I had set goals before I met Jack. There were things I wanted to achieve, and I took the steps to get there. The difference is I never really thought of them as goals, and I didn't have a specific plan as to how to achieve them.

When you set out to do something without a specific plan, your objective can seem out of reach, impossible to obtain. But, if you write it down and make a plan for how you are going to get there, all of a sudden the steps are in front of you and the goal seems much easier to attain.

During the summer before my eighth grade year, my goals were the usual eighth grade goals. I wanted to be popular, thin, smart, and have boyfriends, clear skin, and a closet full of clothes, not necessarily in that order. I would dream and think how great it would be if some of those things happened. I had even achieved some of those things, but it was all sort of at random and by accident. I looked at my achievements as a freak accident, as luck. My low self-esteem kept me from believing that I had any control over what would happen to me. As I worked on improving my self-esteem, I realized that I could influence my life if I planned for success and believed it was possible.

I learned to write out all my goals, even the most outrageous, far-out dreams. I had to distinguish between what Jack called, "short term goals and long term goals." My short term goals were clear skin and keeping up my grades. My long term goals for the future were to be a professional singer and author.

Short term goals are things you want to achieve in the near future. I think of short term goals as those things that are a little closer and more accessible. The short term goals are the small steps that lead you to the large goal. For instance, taking singing lessons would be a short term goal because it would help me achieve my long term goal of being a singer someday. Going to school and achieving high grades would be a short term goal because it would help me become an author.

I wrote all my goals down and put the short term and long term goals on two different lists. I put the most important short term and long term goals at the top. Once I had the goals written down, I read them out loud. I was overwhelmed by the things I had written. I wanted to be an author and a singer, things that seemed so far out of reach, and yet there they were. At first, I wanted to crumple up the list as I had done before, throw it away, and continue to believe that these things were impossible. Then I looked at it again and was intrigued by the possibility that if I made a plan and started right now, maybe I could make it.

A year ago, while I was working on this book, I picked up a binder that had been hidden away in a large book shelf for years. I opened the binder and found the goals that I had written in my scrawled handwriting that summer before the eighth grade. To my amazement, almost every one of those goals had come true! Yes, my skin did clear up. The few goals that hadn't been achieved turned out to be things I didn't want anyway. Some of the goals that I had written on those pages took longer than I thought they would to achieve. In fact, some of the goals that I wrote that summer took years to be realized. That is why they were called long term goals. But still, they happened.

Don't crumple up your list. Write your goals down, even the most incredible ones. How could you make those goals happen? How could you put that dream into a plan and make it reality? The short term goals are what will make it happen. Getting out of bed early to go to swim team practice, to study for a test, to practice your instrument, to get ready for school, going to a tutor or going to school early to ask for help; these are all action steps that will help you realize your goals.

You set your goals, make a plan, write it, say it to yourself, take action, and the goals will be attained. I thought Jack was kidding me when he told me about positive thinking. I thought, "You're crazy, Jack, life isn't like that. Things just happen to you." I learned to believe it, to use all the tools I have listed above, and I also learned to combine those tools with a strong faith in God.

Sometimes I lost my way. There were times that I stopped doing all the things that made me feel better and helped me to improve. Sometimes I stopped because I thought, "I am doing so well, I don't need those things anymore," or "I'm doing fine now, I don't need to have a plan." During these times, I would wake up wondering why I felt so lousy, and wonder why I came home from school with my brain swimming in negative self-talk. It was usually at that point that I would remember, "Maybe I should pray about it, go back to my goals, and get on track again."

At the end of this book, you will find a bibliography which may help you with new ideas for building your self-esteem and achieving your goals. I have only listed those books that I have used and found helpful. You may find some on your own that are useful, too. In the process of gathering ideas on any subject through reading, lectures, and tapes, remember to take what you think is valid and disregard the rest. If you go to a lecture and ask yourself, "Was that person for real?" maybe that isn't the information you want to hang on to.

I learned from Jack and my mom that motivational speakers and writers can be a dime a dozen. Some, as in every profession, may not have your best interests in mind. You don't have to spend a lot of money on a book or tape to start thinking positively. The bottom line is that you have to listen to the messages you're sending to yourself. Every person on this earth has a value and a purpose, but you have to feel good about yourself before you can truly discover what that is. You can start anywhere, anytime. All you need is yourself and the will to make a change.

By the time that summer before my eighth grade year had come to an end, I found myself actually looking forward to a new school year rather than dreading it. My mom's health was improving, and she had a good man in her life. I was ready to take on the ninth grade with a positive attitude.

NINTH GRADE

Have you ever gotten fired up about something, forged ahead with gusto, then the flame sort of fizzled out? I held out with my binder and my goal setting for a long time, two months to be exact. Then with the hurry and bustle of school, my time was put into other things.

It is hard to be dedicated to goal setting, studying, practicing, and faith. There always seems to be something better to do. The problem is that if you don't stick to it, you won't see the results.

Slowly but surely, I found myself relying on my old way of living: push, push, push. "You're not good enough! What is the crisis of the day? Why aren't I happy?" That summer I was fired up and ready to goal-set my way to happiness. But when the school year started and some problems arose here and there, instead of praying about it or working on my attitude, I backslid right into my old way of thinking. I could have stopped it, but I just let it happen.

That year was like the others. I was searching again, looking for something that seemed to be missing in myself, some kind of validation which would fill up the empty hole I felt inside. And in the process I lost myself.

It was the first trimester of the year and I already was beginning to get the "I'm not enough" blues. Being co-president of the Pep Club was nothing more than selling buttons and school pennants at lunch time and what's worse, nobody wanted to buy them. Even worse was the dance we put on to raise money for Pep Club. Few people came and if we played anything but hard rock, the tough kids booed us. My co-president and I were friends, and we had all kinds of great ideas for things we could do to raise money for the club, most of which were vetoed by administration. In junior high, your opinion as Pep Club president doesn't carry much clout in the adult world.

By the second trimester of the school year, I had a burning need for a new title. There was nothing to run for so I turned to the next best thing, sports. Okay, here is a girl who hates physical education classes, has a curling iron in her gym locker, has tried out for the girl's track team and the community baseball team and managed to quit due to illness or some other excuse. Where is the logic here?

Now, this part is even better. Of all the sports I could have possibly picked to be a part of, I chose gymnastics, which is literally one of the most difficult sports to get involved in for someone with little or no background in athletics.

You may be asking yourself the same question I ask myself even now. Why? Well, it seemed like the right thing to do. The majority of the people I knew were cheerleaders or were involved in sports or band. I had my grades but that was an isolated achievement. I saw everyone else congregating after school with their team members and forming relationships with other students that I never had. I had friends but often felt like I didn't fit. I thought that by joining a sports team I could be a part of something, be involved, have what those other people seemed to have.

Those are not the best reasons for joining a sport you know nothing about, especially one that can be potentially dangerous if you don't know what you're doing. I went with it anyway.

A couple of my friends were trying out for the gymnastics team so we went to the tryouts together and they helped me with the routines. I knew in the back of my mind that it was a long shot. In fact, it still surprises me that I continued in my efforts.

I practiced at school and at home in our living room. What a sight that must have been! My long legs flying through the air, barely missing a lamp or stereo. Although I was in ninth grade, I was trying out with the beginning floor routine, which was rather embarrassing. I would look around at tryouts and see girls who were two years younger than I doing the same routine perfectly while I struggled through.

I went to the tryouts and somehow got through my routine. The girls cheered me on which was encouraging, but it was an embarrassing experience none the less. I never did finish the actual acrobatic moves, like the back somersault handstand. My arms were so thin and unmuscular that they buckled under me.

I didn't really expect to make the team, but I spent the weekend after the tryouts worrying about whether I did or not. Monday came and we all went to practice to hear who had been chosen. To all of our amazement, the coaches announced nobody had been cut from the team.

The coach said that although not everyone was on the competitive team, nobody had been cut from the group. She was a new coach that year and wanted to see what all of us had to offer and what a little practice time would do for some of us. I was relieved I hadn't been cut and at the same time I didn't know what was the point of staying. My tolerance for frustration had already hit an all time high during the tryouts, and I couldn't imagine what it would be like to go to the gym every day and continue practicing.

I wanted it and didn't want it at the same time. I knew early on this wasn't the sport for me, but to save face, I stuck with it. I think I felt that because I hadn't stuck with baseball or track, someone might think that I was a quitter if I dropped off the team.

Though I was right about my lack of ability in gymnastics, there are some things you don't even know you are good at unless you try. I found that was true with singing. If my mom hadn't asked me, I wouldn't have known for many years, or maybe for my entire lifetime, that I could sing. To say that trying out for a sports team was a waste of time for someone else would be wrong. There were girls who tried out for our team with little or no experience who found a talent for gymnastics they didn't know they possessed.

Trying is never wrong.

But I didn't join the team to look for hidden talent. I joined just for acceptance and a new group of friends. I wanted to be somebody and thought a letter on my jacket would be the way.

Instead of spending my time looking for something I would be good at, or spending my time with more studying, dance classes, or singing lessons, I wasted several months in an activity I didn't even like.

I was hurt several times, twice trying a back handspring and later jumping off the beam onto an old spotting block which had a hole in it. My foot went through and twisted. I was on crutches for a week and my ankle is still weak due to that accident. I wasn't doing myself any favors by staying on the team when I really didn't enjoy it. Because I wasn't competing, it was easy to become careless and joke around on dangerous equipment. I'm lucky I didn't come out of this experience with more than just a swollen ankle and a lump on my head.

My only shining moment of this whole experience was when, at the last minute, I was asked to fill in for an injured team member at a meet. I was so thrilled that within minutes I had borrowed a leotard and was warming up. I'd be doing the beginning beam routine. Most of the students I would be competing against were one or two years younger, this routine was as it says, for beginners.

The most difficult part of the routine was a forward roll on the beam. It sounds simple enough, doesn't it, except for the fact that you have to fit your whole body on a board only a few inches wide. Have you ever balanced your head on a board and then tried to roll your whole body over it? It isn't as easy as Olympic gymnasts make it look on television.

I had worked and worked on this routine. I didn't think I would ever compete with it, but I tried anyway. In fact, it was after my first completed forward roll on the beam that I jumped off the beam and fell through the hole in the spotting block. My completing a forward roll was something to cheer about.

When it came my turn at the meet, I went through all the motions. I nodded to the judge, put my hands in the air, flexed my back, and walked toward the beam. I was to run, jump on a spring board, and land with one foot on the beam and one foot off in a squatting position. I was so nervous that I almost overshot the beam and landed on the other side, but I gripped with my toes to hang on. I felt the team's victory or loss hung in the balance so I gripped even tighter.

I could feel the audience looking at me. Oh, yes, it must be me, or maybe it's the three other people doing floor, bars, and vault exercises. Well, anyway, I was nervous. I went through all the little ballet motions with a little wobble here, a little wobble there.

The judge was scribbling madly on her clipboard, I could see her out of the corner of my eye.

Then came the most important part of the routine, the dreaded forward roll. At this moment, I self-talked myself through the task, but still my legs shook with fear. I lowered my head down, put it on the beam, raised my hips in the air, and started to roll. It started at my feet and went to my head in minutes, the uncontrollable trembling and shaking was starting. I tried to hold my head to the beam, but I was leaning from side to side. All at once I wanted to shout, "Timber!"

I found myself sitting on the floor. I had fallen. I jumped back on the beam and started all over again in the forward roll position. I was determined to make it over and through the forward roll this time. I made it over but just before I had my legs touching the beam I was on the floor again. I started to ask myself, "If you do badly, do they deduct points from other people's score, too?"

When I had done my dismount, I didn't know whether to laugh or cry. Then came the crowning blow. One of the younger girls on the team, who was a born gymnast, came up and said, "Nice exhibition routine."

"What exhibition," I asked?

She said, "You just did an exhibition routine."

I argued with her; then I said, "Wait a minute, what is an exhibition routine?"

"It means that you did your routine, but the score wasn't counted."

Well, that was a rude awakening. I had just publicly humiliated myself, beat myself up against the ground, and jumped several feet in the air on a thin board in front of several hundred people for nothing. It was probably for the better, I think my score was the lowest of the day anyway. But still, why didn't they just tell me it didn't count? Then someone else could have gone up and put themselves through the turmoil. I went home slightly depressed, but now it all seems hilarious. Shari Rusch, a gymnast? Not in this lifetime. I was sad to find out that the only people who got letters for being on the gymnastics team were those who actually competed. What kind of deal is that?

I was totally disgusted with myself for having held out on a team, then didn't even get a letter. Actually, it served me right, I was searching and came up empty handed. If I had just stopped looking so frantically, I would have saved myself time, energy, and a twisted ankle. Getting a letter or a spot on a team was just a filler, not the answer.

Within a few weeks of the gymnastics season being over, I found out that the high school was going to be having tryouts for a new junior varsity cheer squad. I wanted to kick myself, this is what

I had really wanted to do all along. The amazing thing was that I had written in my goal book that I wanted to be cheerleader the next year. The problem was that there was no such thing as sophomore cheerleaders at our local high school. I wrote that goal during the summer, and eight months later they decided to have a junior varsity cheer squad at the high school for the first time.

Someone once said, "Be careful what you ask for, you might actually get it." As I said before, everything I set goals for that summer, even those goals that were a long way off, happened.

Use your time wisely, on activities you enjoy, and that are good for you. If you try one thing and it doesn't work, try another. But give each thing you try a little time. You may start out not doing well and within a period of time develop a knack for it.

Most of all, know that God has a timing for things. Sometimes it doesn't fit our time schedule, sometimes you have to work and labor without reward for a while, and then the plan will be clearer to you as you go along. If I had worked to improve myself in areas that were positive rather than searching blindly in everything and anything, I could have saved myself some trouble and in a few months the plan would have been clear. When you push things, it usually doesn't get you there any faster, just with more mistakes.

CHEERLEADING

I learned from my experience with gymnastics. When I heard the news about tryouts for cheerleading, I decided to do things differently than before. I decided to make a goal out of cheerleading. Maybe my motivation was the same as it had always been; I wanted to be popular, I wanted a group to belong to, and an activity to be involved in. But this meant more to me because I had to wait for it. The year before had brought its disappointments and now I had a chance to try again.

Considering I had no experience in cheerleading and very little in dance, I knew it would require a lot of practice to make it on a cheer squad. A position on the junior varsity cheer squad became the goal. Constant practicing, and goal setting became my strategy for success.

My partner and I practiced until every muscle in our bodies was sore. My friend had cheerleading experience at our junior high school, so she already knew what she was doing. I, on the other hand, just had natural rhythm. The rest I had to work on. I had never done straight arm moves like they were teaching us at the high school during rehearsals. I thought my arms would break off if I held them any stiffer, but I kept working.

Even when I was too tired to practice anymore, visualizing the cheers or dance in my head served as another way to get the information to stick.

My greatest problem occurred when I went to the tryout rehearsals up at the high school. I found myself doing a majority of the moves backwards. The varsity cheerleaders who were teaching us our routines would put their hands to the right; I put my hands left. They would step left; I would step right. I would squint my eyes, even move myself to the front, but I still found it was hard to get the information through my eyes and filtered out to my arms and legs correctly. The pressure of wanting to do it well only made it worse.

Cheerleading was much like riding a bike for me, I couldn't seem to put everything together at once. Each of my arms, legs, hands, and feet seemed to work independently of each other. My eyes, which were taking in the information, couldn't seem to store the information in the right order, and compute which direction the move should go.

To learn a cheer I had to watch someone do it, follow their hands, feet, arms, and body moves in motion to a rhythm. I also had to say the words to the cheer in order and make them correspond to the right moves. While doing all of this, I was to smile, jump and look totally at ease. Just as my brain overloaded while I tried to learn how to ride a bike, it also overloaded while I was cheering.

Learning the cheers took constant repetition, as with everything else in my life. In time, I found the words and pattern of the cheer, once learned, actually became my study guide. Each move had a word, each word had a move. Each thing I did had something to go with it, which helped me make the connection. It was like learning a song. I could learn a song because of its pattern and its repetition. The cheers, too, had a pattern and repetition which helped me to learn and remember them.

This experience reminded me, just in case I might have forgotten, that it was possible for me to be good at athletics, dance, and other physical activities; but like my studying, it would require another form of learning.

My mind and body may have not been connected very well, but they were connected. It was just a matter of seeing which way I could learn best. Was it seeing someone do it facing me or with their back to me? Did I need it broken down or in its regular rhythm and pattern? Would I prefer learning it with the words, without the words, with only the arms first and then adding the feet, with a mirror or without a mirror, what? I figured it out and learned the cheers and the dance I would need to try out with in ninth grade. To this day, I am still using those strategies to learn dance routines for a show or for a dance class.

At first, I was highly frustrated; I would just learn something and then it would be gone. I would remember the words to the cheer but not the moves, remember the move just not the direction. As much as I hated it, I became very good at asking for help. I knew that it was either ask or not try out.

There were days that I would come home from practice and drop on the couch in exhaustion. Even when I was tired, my mind would still be focused on my goal. I would be drifting off to sleep or daydreaming, and in my mind's eye I could almost see the cafeteria where we would be trying out. I saw all the judges sitting in their chairs with the judging forms in front of them and all the contestants sitting in their chairs nervously. I on the other hand, sat calmly in my chair as if I didn't have a care in the world.

In my daydream, I hear my name being called and I take the floor. I see myself doing every cheer in order, without a single mistake. I see myself dancing through our dance as if it was the easiest thing I have ever done. I smile, I charm, I have the judges in the palm of my hand. Then, when I am finished with the dance, I jump so high I almost touch the ceiling and yell so loud nobody else can be heard. The judges jump to their feet and come up to me with a black and gold sweater in their hands and say in a sugary sweet way, "Shari, will you please, please be a junior varsity cheerleader?"

And I look at them and say, "Well, if I can find the time." Why dream anything but the best?

Jack used to tell me to set your sights for more than what you want, rather than less. That way there is no room for doubt. My goal to be a cheerleader seems a little far out now, but at the time, it was such an important goal in my life that I tried hard to think positively about it.

When the big day came, nobody came up to me and begged me to be on the cheer squad or handed me a cheer sweater as I had imagined they would. Maybe I didn't jump as high as in my dreams, but I did better that day than I had ever done in my life, in anything that had to do with athletics or dancing that is. There is no question in my mind that working hard, setting my goals, and thinking positive helped.

I made the squad! I don't want to sound dramatic, but it changed my life at that moment. To be accepted into that circle was similar to being asked to be in honors English and Social Studies; all of a sudden I was validated and accepted. For that moment, when my name was announced, it was like a butterfly coming out of her cocoon. I raised up my shoulders and walked a little prouder. I believed in myself, and I reached my goal. Now I got to see what it was like on the other side of the fence.

Reaching a goal really is like going to the other side of a fence. We've been looking over that fence and we think that people on the other side have it all. But when we get to their spot, we sometimes see that the grass isn't always greener on the other side.

THE OTHER SIDE OF THE FENCE

Being on the other side of the cheerleading fence was different from what I had expected. It was much like the feeling of getting straight A's and then realizing that I now had to try to keep them. The amount of time I had spent trying to become a cheerleader, learning that one cheer and one dance, left me wondering if I would have to do that for every cheer. Yes, for a while that was so. I wanted to waltz in and feel the glamour of the position, but when it's 8:00 in the morning every day of the week during the summer, and you have practice for two hours, and you spend that two hours struggling to learn, cheerleading loses its glitter very quickly.

But that was just the beginning. I found out quickly that cheer squads can have cliques, too. Just because you are on the squad, a member of the team, or a member of the club doesn't mean that people have to accept you. It just means that you work with each other. The ideal experience that I had envisioned wasn't what I got.

From the beginning, I didn't feel I belonged. I was looking for a group to accept me and instead found myself on the outside. Sometimes others put me there, sometimes I put myself there because I didn't know how to relate to or be a part of a group. I had never had a group to belong to before!

But I could overlook all these things because this was the first year my sister and I had attended a school together when I didn't feel like an embarrassment to her. Sadly enough, I thought that my sister had spent most of her life being embarrassed of me and what other kids said or thought about me. I felt that for me to be at the same school as her, I needed to be her equal. I thought by being a cheerleader I would be.

STUMBLING BLOCKS TO STEPPING STONES

CHAPTER 15

CHANGES

Just prior to my sophomore year, my mom and Jack broke up. By this time, my mom was almost completely healed from her illnesses, she and Jack had started a highly successful singles group called TLC, and both were doing well in their business endeavors. Even with everything going so well, I could tell that their relationship was coming to an end.

They parted still caring and respecting each other, and they remain friends to this day. This made it easier for me to adjust to another change. I took all the good advice and friendship that Jack had given me, and I was glad he had come into our lives.

Not long after my mom broke up with Jack, she began seeing a man named Rod Pressey. He was the activities coordinator and basketball coach at our high school and had substituted as cheer advisor during my sister's first year on the high school cheer squad.

Shawn grew fond of him when he was her cheer advisor and she kept saying, "Mom, you ought to date someone like Mr. Pressey." She would always come home with mention of him. Mr. Pressey this, Mr. Pressey that, and when my Mom visited our school, my sister introduced them.

A year after their first meeting, they met again during the summer before my sophomore year. By October of that year, less than three months after meeting each other for a second time, they were married.

All of it happened so fast that I didn't really have time to cope with the idea. We were just two years past a nightmare. Who would want to go through that again, and yet, who wouldn't want Mr. Pressey as their stepfather? I couldn't help but like Rod, but I was still afraid.

My sister sort of threw up her hands. She was happy for them but, like me, was a little scared. I gave them my blessing, but shook in my boots. Even my mom said she almost called the whole thing off the night before the wedding because she was so frightened. She had to have been thinking, "Am I making another mistake?" She wasn't. Rod is a wonderful man and they still love each other very much after almost 10 years of marriage. But all of us were nervous then.

It was at a football game that I found out that my mom and Rod were engaged. One of Rod's fellow educators took the microphone up in the press box at the stadium where our high school played and announced the engagement to the whole crowd. When the announcement was made, I had already left the stadium with some of my friends and was at a pizza parlor up the street. Within minutes all my friends came in telling me the good news. When you have loud friends, who needs a microphone!

237

During the ceremony, Rod gave Shawn and me wedding rings, and my mom gave his two children wedding rings to signify all of us joining together. I wore that ring until my own marriage.

BLENDING

Even though Rod had two grown children of his own, he chose to be a father to my sister and me. He could have been scared off by two teenage daughters, but he wasn't.

I don't know if my sister needed a father in the same way I did or if she was even looking for one. She was older and more in control of her life. She had the contact with my father that I had never had. I was the one who needed a father figure.

As much as I wanted to attach myself to Rod, I feared another loss. And as much as he wanted to reach out to me, he was unsure how to do it without being pushy. His personality was quiet and subdued, and I kept myself at a distance, not wanting to commit myself to anything. I was afraid to trust Rod for fear he'd leave me. I didn't want to set myself up for a disappointment. I thought that if I started to need him, then he could disappoint me. If I stayed distant, I was untouchable.

I wasn't quite sure what to think of Rod's quiet manner. I was used to people using silence as means of control and anger. He didn't have an angry bone in his body; however, because he didn't talk like a chatter box, I was afraid that there was something wrong or that he was upset with me. Many times I went crying to my mom and said, "What's wrong with Rod; are you going to get a divorce?" or "Is he mad at me?"

She would calmly reassure me and say, "No, everything is just fine, that's just his way. He is quiet, not unhappy or angry." Even with all the reassurance, even with all the love and caring that Rod showed, it was still hard for me to accept that his love was real and he wasn't going to leave us.

At the same time that I was trying to adjust to a new stepfather and a new living situation, I also started dating. I was beginning to feel the effects of having an absentee father, though I wasn't aware of the cause of my feelings at the time. I had tried to form a relationship with my first stepfather, but that didn't work. I had done the same with my mom's boyfriends, but they were not permanent relationships. I even tried to start a relationship with my new stepfather. I needed Rod's love, but I couldn't face the possibility of losing another father. When I reached age fifteen or sixteen, I made an unconscious decision to look elsewhere for the love I needed.

Without realizing it, I started to look at relationships with people my own age as being the way to provide me with value and self-worth. If a boy liked me, I felt that I was receiving the approval that I had always wanted. This approval seemed to be safe. The truth is, depending on someone besides yourself to give you worth is never safe.

I began a pattern in my relationships early on. I tended to choose people who were less than what I may have deserved because I didn't think I deserved any better. I also chose people who needed me to take care of them. I figured if they couldn't take care of themselves, they wouldn't leave me. I had watched my mom and my sister have the same type of relationships, now it was my turn. Not every relationship in their lives was like that, but there was a definite trend. My mom had broken the cycle with Rod, but my sister and I still didn't realize what we were doing.

I perceived boys and men to be better than me. Because I was so desperate for love, I allowed people to hurt my feelings, let me down and use me, all the while thinking that without that person, I was nothing.

I wish Rod had come into our lives sooner; I know his love could have saved me from many mistakes. But ultimately, it was those mistakes and bad choices in relationships that helped me to understand why the kids I speak to do what they do.

I remember not long after my mom and Rod were married and we had moved into Rod's house, I asked a senior to a dance. A sophomore ask a senior! I still can't believe I had the nerve, but I had a crush on this guy so big it could have touched the sky. One time I was walking down a walkway at school watching him walk. I was so absorbed in watching him that I ran right into a pole. Now, that's a crush! We dated for a few weeks and then it was over. I was devastated beyond belief. I thought, as we all do at one time or another, that I would never find someone like him.

The day he broke up with me, I came home from school and played every sad song I owned on my record player. It was February, the rain was falling and the fog was rolling in. The perfect setting for a broken romance. Rod came in, put his arm around me and said, "Shari, if you ever need to talk to anyone, you can always come to me." I wanted to reach out and hug him, to take from him all the love that I knew that he had to give me, but I held myself back. I gave him a little hug, but it was forced. I told him that I would come to him in the future, but I knew deep inside I wouldn't be able to.

Fortunately, Rod was a very patient person. Because he didn't come rushing in and try to smother me, I could get used to the idea of trusting a man and was able to come to him on my own terms. On the other hand, because he wasn't aggressive and left it up to me, I found myself unable to get very close to him. I didn't know how.

Just hugging him made me feel afraid and very vulnerable. Just like some people are afraid to cry, to show emotion or to say I love you, I was afraid that after I opened myself up to him that my vulnerability would be used against me. Maybe that's the legacy of divorce. I learned to be afraid and distrustful. I was making decisions according to the past, and it ruined what could have been a loving father-daughter relationship.

Even though my relationship with my father was poor at this point, I still clung to it and couldn't let go. I wouldn't allow myself to love Rod like a father. I thought I was doing the right thing - showing loyalty to my father no matter what. I didn't want to disassociate myself from my father, nor would I allow someone else to love me in his place.

I continued in my search for love and acceptance. No cheer sweater, straight A average, or two week romance would satisfy my need. My two week romances seemed harmless; none of them lasted long enough to create any serious problems. But I was getting older. In books and magazines and around every corner, I saw people who seemed to be in love. Now that I was older, I wanted to fall in love. I guess I was looking for a missing piece of me that I thought I would find in someone else. I thought that if a boy loved me, then it could fill up the emptiness in my life, and replace anything that was missing.

I could write a book on this subject alone. I meet girls and boys who go through these same feelings, but the difference is that so many of them end up pregnant or as young fathers. Why did they do it? A lot of them just wanted love.

SINGING

In my search to find acceptance and love, I stumbled back into something that I had left behind so many years before.

I can remember when I was in fifth grade I would come home after school to an empty house. After cleaning the house top to bottom, I would walk downstairs and sit on the floor next to our record player, put on a record, and sing until my voice was hoarse. By fifth grade, I seldom performed in public. I was shy and far too critical of myself to stand on a stage. Whether I would sing in public or not, I never stopped singing when I was alone.

At eleven, sitting in front of that record player, I would perform. I didn't play pop tunes like other children my age, I played Barbra Streisand, her early records particularly. One record was my favorite. It was a live album, Barbra Streisand at the Forum. I would sing "Stony End," "People," "My Man," and all her other wonderful songs. Most kids that age probably would have found the lyrics hard to understand, but not me. I was so old at eleven, I could easily relate to the words.

I would play parts of that live album over and over again for one and only one reason, I wanted to hear the applause. I sang with Barbra Streisand, and then I would bask in the applause from the live album as if it was for me.

At sixteen, I started singing again because I wanted love. I thought that the applause in the audience would fill me up and heal my pain. A few months into my sophomore year, I signed up for a talent show at school. I dressed as a barmaid and sang, "I Didn't Know the Gun was Loaded," my childhood theme song, and a medley of songs from the musical, Annie.

People were surprised. Shari sings? I was surprised at myself. The fear inside me was so great, but it was worth every bit of it when I heard the applause. It was another type of recognition, a kind that I hadn't experienced in a long time.

From that talent show on, I decided I wanted to sing again. I didn't know where or when, I just knew that I couldn't live without the feeling that comes when people applaud for you. I craved that feeling. For in that moment, no matter how fleeting, I felt like I was somebody.

In many regards singing became a love hate relationship for me. I loved the applause, but I was so afraid of making a mistake, of being vulnerable, of being criticized by anyone including myself that it was hard to enjoy the rewards. I loved singing, and I wanted to be good at it. But how do you become good when you are so afraid of making a mistake, you can barely take the stage?

The first time that I sang again, I realized that Rod's opinion of how I had done was most important of all. He was my father by then, I needed him to tell me what I needed to hear. I needed to be enough for him. Rod learned very early to say something to me right away when he saw me after a performance. If he smiled, it wasn't enough. If he said, "Good job," it still wasn't enough. Because my father had never acknowledged my performances very much, a man's opinion was the most frightening.

Eventually, singing would be an effortless way for me to express myself. But at this point in my life I was so hungry for praise, so eager to find my value in the world, that even a joyous moment was circled with doubt. In everything that I did, I begged for praise.

By the time I got to my senior year, I was a classic overachiever. I had it all, as they say, but I always felt empty. I literally almost lost my mind in the battle to be the best and hide any imperfection from the world. Let me explain the sequence of events that led me to the state I was in during my senior year.

CHEERLEADING

To stay on a cheer squad I had to work overtime to learn the cheers. Granted, it was only a junior varsity cheer squad for the first year in high school, so the pressure was less intense. But it took me so long just to learn a cheer, one cheer, that by the end of the first year, I was exhausted.

I had vowed I would never let anyone see my differences. Both at practice and games, I tried to pretend that I knew the cheers and dances just like everyone else. In time, it became obvious that I was not like everyone else. People became used to actually taking me by the shoulders and moving me into position because I couldn't ever remember what direction I was supposed to go or which position I had in the line. It was almost funny. I became used to asking people to stay after school to go over a cheer with me one more time. I became used to it, but I still found it embarrassing to ask for help from people my own age.

The need for help became even greater when I was selected for the varsity cheer squad in my junior year. Now there were a hundred cheers to learn and so little time. Fortunately, some of the older girls on the squad offered me help which saved me from embarrassment, but it was still hard to keep up.

Some would say, "Well, Shari, why didn't you just tell the girls what the problem was." No, I don't think so. I had worked all my life to hide my differences, I wasn't going to start revealing them now. I learned to handle the fact that I was prone to mistakes by making fun of myself, calling myself an airhead or a dumb blonde. I thought that being a dumb blonde was better than being learning disabled.

Others ask, "Why didn't you quit?" I wouldn't have quit no matter what. As I look back on it, cheerleading was more of a hassle than it was fun, but there were moments at games when the feeling was so great. It was the feeling that singing gave me; I was somebody.

It's like asking me, "Why did you continue to get good grades? You've proved it is possible, now ease up on yourself." That wasn't the way it was for me; the grades were me now. The report card and cheer sweater were my value, to give them up would mean I was nothing. I looked in the mirror in sixth grade and despised what I saw. I would look at other people and think, "Why can't I be like them?" By late junior high and high school I had become them on the outside, but on the inside I still felt like a resource room kid. I still whipped myself with the words, "You aren't good enough." Once I made it, I had to stay. Once I stayed, I had to have more.

MATH PROBLEMS

The pressure from school was enormous. I knew when I started

242

high school it would be very hard for me. I was right; the work was harder, the work load greater, and on top of that, I had the responsibility and time commitment of cheerleading.

At the beginning of my sophomore year, I signed up for a math teacher who was highly recommended. Why wouldn't he be recommended? He was a whiz at math and computer science. He was the genius that people told me he was, but they left one thing out: he didn't have much time for a slow student like myself.

He was nice, so I thought we could work it out. But his eyes said, "If you don't understand, why are you in the class?" He was smart, and all the other smart students sat in his class and nodded their heads while he skipped over steps and painted broad strokes over a problem that I needed to have dissected.

The schedule of events in his class was very strange. We would take a quiz and then go over the previous day's lesson and homework. Although there was time to ask questions prior to the quiz, it was never enough. The teacher moved quickly, talked quickly, and his eyes urged me to hurry and finish what I was saying because he had more important things to do. I cannot learn in this way.

I found myself floundering in his class from the very start. I tried to get help during work time, but he was always in a hurry. I went in after school, but he was either working on the computers with his computer students or going off to a sports event at school. In his haste, I was failing. I was doing as I always had done - trying to stay in the class, doing whatever I had to do to get extra help - and still I was not doing well.

It got so bad that at one point, I went up to the teacher after everyone had left the room. I said, "Prior to entering your class, I was an A student. I have learning disabilities and have to work extremely hard to get that kind of grade. I am now at a C in your class and dropping quickly. I desperately need help or I'm going to drop out of the class." He assured me that this was only the second test and he would give me more time. I asked him if it was possible for me to get an A from the class, and he said that it was. He said he would help me.

I never did get that help. As well intentioned as he was, he was split in too many directions. He had a full load of math classes, he was a coach, and he was teaching computer classes. After our talk, I went in after school expecting that he would feel some responsibility to me now that I was staying in his class, but instead I received a few fleeting moments of instruction which was usually interrupted by him leaving the room to answer a question from one of his other students. Sometimes I would go to his room and receive no instruction at all. He just didn't have the time.

The worst part for me was that I felt trapped. I might have been able to transfer classes early when I first went to him with my problems in the class. I had already talked to my counselor and she would have made the arrangements. In a hurried manner he told me to stay, and we would work it out. I couldn't work it out alone, which is what ended up happening.

I can sympathize. We are all human, over-booking ourselves at times and making promises that are hard to keep. But in the process of being busy, my teacher was giving me only one ear to hear my problems and only one hand, if any, to help me. Because of this, I was going to get a B in his class and break my straight A record for the first time in four years.

I thought my teacher was a good man, but he made me feel helpless. I couldn't do it without him, but he was never there. There were some things that I could do on my own, but I learned very early that I needed teachers to teach me. I depended on them.

Depending on people made me feel extremely helpless. If I had a teacher who took the time for me, I felt confident about my abilities. But when I had a teacher who couldn't give me some individual instruction, I felt dependent and felt I would always be one step behind those who didn't have learning disabilities.

I had come to believe that without my grades I was nothing. With that attitude, the B I received in that math class may as well have been an F. It's hard to understand this, unless you realize the struggle it took for someone like me to achieve the A's that I had earned before. I was angry at myself for showing that I might not be perfect, and for needing so much help all the time. But I was even more angry at my helplessness in the world.

Wanting to prove everyone wrong was not why I had originally tried to do well in school, but it had come to that now. I made a solemn vow that I would never get another B again.

DRIVING

When I went back to school after Christmas vacation of my sophomore year, I found my next test waiting. Such a simple thing, learning how to drive. Everyone learns to drive and gets a license. My sister went on her birthday and passed the test. I thought, "How hard can it be?" My birthday was January 21, and I was determined to go in and take that test if it was the last thing I did.

They say that learning how to drive comes naturally, kind of like riding a bike. Do you remember the bike story I told earlier? Well, now think of it in terms of a large motor vehicle on the roads moving at 55 miles per hour. Frightening, isn't it?

I took Drivers Education and passed all the written tests and book work. Then came the tough part, getting in the car and driving. My car had two male students with a male teacher. I received a clear message from them about their estimation of my driving ability when both of the male students went out on the highways and side streets to learn how to drive, but the teacher took me back to the school to drive in the parking lot.

Our teacher wasn't being sexist, he was just being smart. I had very little sense of direction. I tended to get right and left mixed up. My eye-hand-foot coordination had never been good and my reaction time was slow, neither of which helped my driving skills.

My mom would say a silent prayer every time I went out to drive with someone. She wouldn't ride with me. Two dyslexics in a car is not a good idea. My sister was very grateful that she wasn't old enough to ride with me. My stepbrother was over once and determined very quickly that I shouldn't drive a stick shift; we both had whiplash when the ride was over. I think my stepbrother was glad he lived a great distance away from us after that. Then there was my stepdad, God bless him. Rod was the only one with enough patience to teach me. Our lessons were few and far between because he was extremely busy, but he helped me learn and didn't yell, "Look out!" like my mom did.

Even with help it would take me many more months, even years, to learn how to drive. Driving a car was like being under constant pressure. Pressure was what made my mind short circuit. It's what made me drive through stop lights and signs, miss turn-offs and speed limit change signs, roll over curbs, back into fences, and generally drive like Mr. Magoo.

If driving wasn't such a serious thing, this whole story would be funny. People like me do not always have trouble driving, but those of us who do can attest to the fact that it's a struggle like no other to judge distance, speed, turns, gauges, pedals, obstacles, and everything else inside a metal case, with a hood you can't see beyond.

A few days after my birthday, with my Drivers Education certificate in hand, my grandmother took me to take my test. I passed the written test with a score of 82. I was scared to take it, but they allowed as much time as you needed. I just took a deep breath and went for it.

I scheduled an appointment for the driving part of the test and once again my grandmother accompanied me to the Division of Motor Vehicles. I didn't tell everyone at school what I was doing. I was scared that if I didn't pass, I would have to tell everyone what happened.

The first omen that all would not go well was that one of the blinkers on our car was broken. They checked all the signals, then told me I couldn't take the test with a broken blinker. I was worried, but Grandma was able to fix it by pinching a few wires in the trunk.

Once we were in the car, I felt this terrible rush of adrenaline.

People say to use that adrenaline to help you. Right. When you have a lady sitting next to you staring at every single move you make, you don't think, "Gee, I think I'll use this fear to my benefit." My hands shook so much when I put on my seat belt I couldn't get the tongue into the buckle. I struggled and struggled with it until finally I heard a click. I kept thinking, "And that was just buckling the seat belt!"

To make a long story short, I hit all the poles I could hit during the parallel parking portion of my test and nearly ran over the curb while backing around it. You name it, I did it. She told me to go left, I went right, just like that. She looked at me like I was crazy, and I thought, "Lady, you haven't seen anything yet." With each move I made, the tester would write something. This was like being back in fourth grade with a sheet of times-tables in front of me. The teacher says, "Go," and my brain goes right out the window.

We were headed back to the Department of Motor Vehicles office when I heard the tester yelling, "Stop!" By now I was so scared, my brain so frazzled with stress, I couldn't think straight. I heard her yelling and at that point my mind short circuited. I wanted to hit the brake pedal but instead hit the gas and went right through a stop sign. As I saw the stop sign go by, I figured that I probably wouldn't be getting my license that day. I was right.

I have had teacher after teacher, especially those who work with learning disabled students, thank me for telling my infamous driving story. Many learning disabled kids fail their first driving test. I know kids who have flunked their drivers test time and time again. They know how to drive and are good at it, but their skills are hidden by the pressure of the testing situation.

A drivers license is your rite-of-passage at sixteen whether you are learning disabled or not; but if you are learning disabled, the actual test to get your license becomes just another struggle in the uphill battle of trying to survive in a world with a brain that works differently. You want that license but are afraid to fail; if you do fail, you are afraid to tell anyone.

When I went back to school after my test people asked, "Did you get it?" I couldn't tell them the truth.

I said, "No, I couldn't take the test, my blinker broke. Yes, that's it, my blinker broke." You think that's a dumb answer? They believed it. I didn't want people to think I was stupid or incapable, so I lied.

I didn't go in to try for my license again for another six months. I feared driving and felt I would never be good at it. What an awful feeling that was. While my friends were driving all over the place, I was hiding another secret from the world.

I made up one excuse after another when asked when I would get my license. After the blinker story wore off, I had to come up with other stories. Lying about why I didn't have a license didn't feel very good, but I felt that telling the truth would be worse. I refused to admit to myself or others that I had failed. I didn't even tell my sister for a long time. I never told my boyfriend or even any of my closest friends.

Six months later I went in to take the test again. As I waited in the car for the tester to come out and join me, I was more than surprised when the same tester that I had before walked out of the building and over to my car. She looked more panicked than I felt.

She checked all my signal lights, then got in the car. She got in but left one foot outside the door as if she wanted to leave an out for herself. She asked me if I had any problem with her testing me again and I said, "No." She looked a little disappointed but took a deep breath, pulled her foot in the car and shut the door.

I passed the test that time with only a few minor errors, but it would be a long time before I would drive without any problems. A few months later, just a few blocks from my home, I misjudged the signal that a car in front of me was making and in the process I hit the car, knocking that car's fender down the street. As I watched the owner of the car go to retrieve his fender from down the street, I didn't know whether to laugh or cry.

The driving stories I have would curl your hair. Not because I drive wildly, in fact I drive like a granny behind the wheel. I have had people honk, wave, and do everything but set their clothes on fire to get my attention, but to no avail. Once I'm behind the wheel, I'm in a different time warp.

Oh yes, I concentrate hard on what I'm doing, but still I make mistakes. I make mistakes when I'm in a hurry, under pressure, lost, or listening to the radio, which is just about all the time. It's getting better, but my mom still won't ride with me and I've been driving for years now. That's okay, I won't ride with her, either. If we do have to drive together, she drives, we get lost, and I yell, "Look out," all the time. Have you ever been on Mr. Toad's Wild Ride at Disneyland? If so, that will give you the feel of what it's like to get in a car with my mom and me.

I can laugh about it now, but at the time I was feeling beaten and embarrassed. God forbid there is something that Shari can't do. Somehow I found a way to cover it up, lie, and hide it. Other people could flunk their driving test, but not me. No, flunking meant I wasn't good enough once again, so I better work hard to make up for my failure. A driver's test, a B, struggling on a cheer squad, struggling to fit in at school, and wanting to have a relationship with my father, all combined to make me feel inadequate and embarrassed of myself.

BURNOUT

This was the beginning of what I call my burnout. It slowly crept up on me like a huge shadow.

Rod once said to my mom, "Shari is one of the saddest kids I've ever seen." My mom told me that she felt her most important goal during my high school years was to make sure I didn't fall apart.

People were watching the burnout happen. I could feel it happening, too, but I couldn't prevent it. I would cry myself to sleep with fears and worries of life's simplest challenges. It wasn't just the big things anymore, it was everything. The amazing thing was that even though I was breaking up inside, I would pull myself together in the morning, slap on a smile, and face the day as if nothing was wrong.

The people around me - teachers, friends, and other kids at school - would see the facade and think it was all so easy for me. Some must have wondered if I was human. I would never let anyone see my pain. No one ever saw me break down. I always had a smile on my face, which made some wonder how I could possibly be happy all the time.

I thought I was becoming what people wanted me to be. Didn't they always say, "You're not good enough," or "If you were like us, then we would like you"? Or was it me who said those things? Whether it was someone else or me that set the standard, no matter what I did, I never felt like I reached it.

My way of dealing with that pressure to achieve and fit a mold, was to go in the opposite direction. I reached a point during my junior year where I realized that I wasn't ever going to be "like" anyone else. It was then that I decided to move way from those who didn't understand me or saw me only as the person I was on the outside. It seemed like the only way to survive. I was tired of making fun of myself to fit in, and tired of hiding my differences. In general, I was just tired.

I began isolating myself right after my junior year. By my senior year, I cheered at all the games I was supposed to, did my school work, and made it to school everyday; but that was all. I didn't socialize with anyone if I could help it. I had tried to put up a half-hearted effort, but soon I found the labor of it too great. It was so much easier to be alone.

I found myself more and more tired. My stamina for late nights and early mornings with my books was fading. As my emotional state deteriorated, so did my ability to concentrate and keep up with school. Surprisingly enough, I was able to maintain my average through the first trimester of my senior year. I was second in my class at the time with only one B on my record since junior high.

I thought I could make it, but I could tell that something was happening to me. I was falling asleep with my books and was distracted in class. All of my symptoms of dyslexia were coming out again, everywhere. I was slowly losing control.

I had been the master of control for so long. Do you know what it is like to feel you are losing your grip? None of the tricks were working anymore, and day by day I watched myself slip. I found that all my schoolwork, in fact just going to school, was tedious and exhausting. This feeling that I was slipping only made my fear of failure greater, my need to achieve higher. I worked harder but found myself making less progress.

As I see it now, I needed to stop right then and there to save myself from what was coming. I was on overload but didn't know it; I was showing signs of a breakdown but couldn't see my way clear to stop. In fact, instead of stopping, I just found more ways to overwork myself.

I see the signs so clearly now. The lack of concentration, feeling out of control emotionally, sleeplessness, overwork, exhaustion, fatigue, chronic colds - doesn't it make you tired? It makes me tired to think back on that time. These were my signs of burnout, emotional distress, possibly even a nervous breakdown.

WHAT DO I WANT?

When I say I began isolating myself, I mean I literally removed myself from people and things. In a way I was isolating myself from other people's rejection and opinions, (as well as my own), which was good. But people need people. I had to take the good with the bad. I removed myself from the mainstream, which may have made me lonely, on the other hand it gave me a chance to ask myself, "What do I want to do with my life?"

I was in a confused state at this time. I knew I didn't want to stay where I was and didn't want to go backwards, the only direction left was forward. I just didn't know how to go forward without hurting myself in the process.

THE MOST IMPORTANT GOAL OF ALL

During my junior year, a spokesperson from the Miss America Pageant came to our school and asked several girls, myself included, if we wanted to participate in the local pageant coming up that year. At the time I was too young, but I kept the piece of paper that she gave me and kept the idea in the back of my mind.

At the beginning of my senior year, I sent in an application for the pageant. At the time, it seemed like the perfect way to combine all the things I wanted to do with my life. Most importantly, I thought that as Miss So-and-So I might be able to find the courage to begin talking about my learning problems and maybe people would listen. It never occurred to me that they would listen to me without a title after my name. It felt like the right thing to do at the time, and I plunged into it as I did everything else.

In one sense this was different than everything I had done so far. I wasn't asking for people to accept what I was doing this time. I told few people that I was in the pageant. In this case, and probably for the first time in my life, the goal was mine and the purpose behind it was more important than anything to me, I was finally going to say that I was learning disabled.

When I made the semifinals of the pageant, I realized how much the experience of sitting through modeling classes as a kid, modeling in my mom's fashion shows, and just plain working experience would help me. I had been forced to deal with adults from a very early age and had been performing in some capacity since age five.

While other kids were playing, I had been working. I made my own money and had bought my own clothes for years. Each one of these things prepared me for life and the work I do now; and it certainly helped when I decided to compete in the pageant. I ended up winning the interview and talent contests - and the pageant!

Getting ready for that pageant was nerve wracking, but I can honestly say that during that time was the most balanced period of my whole senior year. Taking my mind off my grades for a little while was exactly what I needed to do. The preparation for the pageant came directly after football season was over, and the pageant was over just before basketball started. I hardly missed a game, and my grades didn't suffer because I was used to doing two activities at once. But again, it was the purpose behind what I was doing that made the goal that much more important and gave me the momentum to achieve like no other goal I had ever set.

I usually dressed up for school, but the day after the pageant, I wore casual clothes. I was unsure of what people would think of me. The announcement that I had won came over the school's loudspeaker in the morning. People I didn't even know came up and congratulated me, others just sort of looked at me wondering when I had done this. Regardless of people's reactions, I thought it was the best day of that whole year. Not because I had won, but because I could feel what it was like to have done something on my own. It was mine.

During my ten-second speech at the pageant, I briefly told of my learning disabilities and said I wanted to be a spokesperson for people like myself. A week after the pageant, I became that spokesperson and gave my first speech at a local Kiwanis group.

When the local papers came to interview me, they picked up on the learning disabilities part of my story. Before I knew it, the city papers were calling to interview me, a story of triumph they called it. I was probably the first dyslexic queen they had ever seen. I'm still surprised that a person like myself who had run away and hidden so well for so long would come out and say, "I am learning disabled." With my parent's support, I started talking.

When I stood before that local Kiwanis group to give my first speech, I recognized people sitting in the audience, a few teachers, even the principal from my school. Telling my story in front of anyone was extremely hard, but it was especially difficult to tell it those educators because I had worked so hard to hide my disabilities from them. But the urgency I felt to let the world know that people like me could make it was greater than the fear.

It had become clear to me that there were millions of people like myself who suffer in silence. Though they graduate from high school, they can't read. They slip through the cracks and slip through life because they don't get proper help for their learning disabilities. I knew of these people long ago, but just didn't have the courage to come forward. I kept wondering, "What will people think, what will they do to me if I tell them?" I had finally arrived at this stage in my life with a near nervous breakdown (and that was with a supportive family). I wondered how other people survived the struggle. That's why I spoke that day. I was almost out of school and had made it, but look at the price I paid.

When my speech was over, I felt relief. There, I had said it! I am learning disabled. The sky hadn't fallen, the world hadn't come to an end, but when I looked out at the audience, the people from my school looked shocked. Some of them were people who had known me for several years, but most didn't truly know me or understand me at all. How can someone be smart, clever, verbal, a cheerleader for goodness sake, and be learning disabled? Why didn't we know this? I could read their minds. It seems ironic that when I went back to school, I was finally able to confront one of them face to face.

After my speech, I went to school a couple of hours late. I entered my third period choir class ten minutes before the bell. I took my seat and watched as students were called up to perform the music they would be doing in an upcoming competition. My teacher had asked me to compete in the competition and had even given me a song to perform, but right before the pageant took place I pulled out of it. I just didn't have enough time.

The minute I sat down, the teacher called to me and said, "Shari, bring your music up and perform your song."

I looked at him rather surprised and said, "I'm sorry, but I'm not prepared".

He looked at me again, and in a stern voice said, "Shari, come up here and perform your song."

I again said, "No, I told you I'm not prepared," then reminded him that I had already told him earlier I was not going to compete. He didn't seem to hear me.

I was feeling the pressure of everyone looking at me and my face was getting hot with embarrassment. My teacher had been known for going off on tirades and throwing tantrums. It was nothing for him to throw his arms up in the air in the middle of a piece of music, storm out of the room slamming his office door behind him, and then not come out for the rest of the class period.

He was a nervous man whose hands were always trembling, and his movements were always quick. His mood swings and intensity made me end up wishing I had never taken the class.

My mind moved quickly, "Was it because I missed most of class this morning?" The second question that entered my mind was closer to the truth, "Was he trying to make an example of me?"

As he kept pressing, his voice became nearly a yell, "Get your music and come up here now!" He had left me no choice. My hands were shaking as I reached for the music in my bag. I realized when I stood up that I still had my heavy coat on. I had been there only minutes when he began pressing me to perform my song. I decided to keep my coat on, though, as if for protection.

I handed him my music and looked up at the clock, wishing for the bell to ring. There were a couple of minutes left of the class as I heard the introduction to my music start. I hated this song. The key was too high and I had told him that. He pointed to the music and looked up, urging me to start the first line. My voice was barely a whisper as the words came out of my mouth. I sang it softly and again looked up at the clock. He saw me look and said, "Keep singing."

He pounded the keys harder and harder, I tried to sing louder but couldn't reach the notes. My voice was tight with tension and there was a lump so big in my throat I thought people must be able to see it from their chairs.

I was near tears as he kept pounding and yelling for me to continue. Each time I stopped to plead with him that I was not prepared to do the song, he would interrupt and say, "Keep going." I could no longer read the words on the page, my mind was tightening as much as my voice.

Everyone sat frozen in their chairs. They couldn't believe what was happening. The bell rang and everyone looked relieved and began to grab their books. I started to walk away from the piano and the teacher yelled, "Everyone stay where you are. She will finish this piece of music. Nobody can leave until she finishes this piece of music."

He said, "Finish it." I thought he must be insane. I was so filled with tears, so humiliated, that nothing would come out now, but he continued to pound away. Finally the song was over and the teacher hit the last notes. I watched as everyone picked up their things and walked away in silence.

I was numb, and the weight of my coat seemed enormous. I was hot with perspiration and embarrassment. I left my sheet music on the piano, walked over to my bag and in one movement, picked it up and walked out the door.

The tears were running down my face and I wasn't about to stop them. I made it only a few steps when a friend stopped me and asked, "Are you okay?"

At first I started to say I was fine, my usual answer. I started to say it, but never finished. I knew that if I walked away then, I always would.

As quickly as I had left, I marched back into the classroom and into my teacher's office. As I blew into the room, some of the students from my choir class were still there and saw how angry I was. It was their first glimpse of Shari Rusch ever losing control of a situation. I walked into my teacher's office and without hesitation, without even saying excuse me, I interrupted his conversation with a student and said, "Could I have a word with you, please?" He saw the look on my face and knew what I was there for.

"How could you do that to me?" I began. "I was not prepared and had even told you I wasn't going to be in the contest, and yet you persisted. You humiliated me in front of people I have worked hard to gain respect from, you embarrassed me in front of my friends."

He came in haltingly, "But Shari, I just thought that you needed a little coaxing, a little push. I thought I needed to encourage you to get up and sing."

Encourage me? That was his idea of encouragement. He knew I would perform anytime if I was prepared. Not long after the pageant he had asked me to perform my pageant song for the class. Without reservation I did it. More than that, he had seen me in the talent shows at school; that's how he knew I could sing in the first place. He knew full well that nobody had to push me.

At that moment, I knew this was just like all the other times I had been made an example. It was either for being too little or too much. This time, I was too much. I walked in with a perfectly matching suit, self-assured, a near straight A student, and cheerleader. From the outside it looked like I had it all, like it was all so easy for me.

I took that moment and said, "Did you know that I have dyslexia? I can't even read your music. As I stood up there under pressure, I couldn't even remember or read the words on the page. Do you know what it's like to be humiliated and embarrassed in front of the people that you have tried all your life to impress? All the people I wanted to like me have now seen me fall apart. Do you have any idea what that is like?" He stood stunned. I said, "I have had to fight to get here, and with one blow you ruined it all."

He said, "Shari, I had no idea."

I said, "That is just the point. You don't know me."

I left his room completely unraveled. When I got home, I was crying so hard that my mom thought I had been in a car accident. I told her the whole story as best as I could in the state that I was in, and she put her arms around me. She told me to go lie down for awhile. I was worried about missing school, but she said that going to school this way was worse than missing. I agreed, and went downstairs to put myself back together again.

When I came back upstairs I found her on the phone talking to my teacher. I immediately panicked, I knew getting mad at him was not going to solve the problem. When I got closer, I could tell that my mom wasn't yelling, or even angry. In a calm voice, she was explaining more about me to my teacher.

When she got off the phone, I was shaking. I was so afraid he would be angry at me for coming in and talking back to him. I usually didn't stick up for myself. The one time I did, I wondered if I did the right thing. My mom assured me that he was sorry about what had taken place and that it wouldn't happen again.

I heard what she said, but I couldn't stop shaking. I felt cold inside, like the world was against me. It had been a long day. I had told my story for the first time and had then been humiliated in class, all in one day. I went back downstairs, shut my door, covered my head with my covers and tried to remove myself from the world with sleep.

CHAPTER 16

COVERING THE PAIN

Sleep had become a remedy for me. I would shut the door to my room and sleep, as a way to shut out my pain. Covered in my blankets, the world could not get to me.

When I was awake, I relied on food to get me through the day. I gained close to thirty pounds by my senior year. Because my bones were so small, I could carry it well. I still wore my cheer skirt and even wore a swim suit in the pageant; it was definitely noticeable, but I could live with it. I knew I had to lose weight for the state pageant. I knew I wanted to lose weight for myself, but I just couldn't seem to do it.

When my insides were cold, food filled the emptiness. Without food in my stomach, I felt I couldn't face the day. Eating was my joy and comfort, and calmed me. It seems strange to use food to fill the void in your life - but food and sleep were like drugs to me.

I had taken a few drinks at parties so that I could feel like one of the crowd; but it made me feel numb and out of control. My drinking never went any further than a few social drinks because while I wanted to be numb, I didn't like the feeling of being out of control. I also knew that if I continued to drink, not only would I lose my self-respect, I would not be able to maintain a straight A average and reach the goals I set for myself. My alternative escape mechanism was to eat. At first I ate because I was hungry, then I ate when I was happy, sad, elated or depressed.

By the second trimester of my senior year, the local pageant was over but the work was just beginning for the state level. I had a full load of classes; I was trying to maintain my grade point, I was still cheering at games, and things were building up. I had personal appearances to make, public speaking to do, preparations for the state pageant, interviews with newspapers and plenty of homework. Somehow I swept through it all without showing my emotions, but when I went home, I would fall apart. I would run fast during the day to keep up and then go home to sleep and eat.

I had been having mood swings and depression for a long time. I thought I had a hormone imbalance or something. By eighteen years old the depression was constant. Like a blanket, it would envelop me from morning to night. It had gone away during the pageant, I had gained a focus and a goal. Christmas vacation had also helped to ease the pressure for a little while. Now I was back at school and my depression returned.

I found myself tired, often sick, and I was cold all the time. I dreaded each day because the cold outside was as cold as I felt inside. From the time I woke up to the time I went to sleep, I was cold. It seemed that it rained every day and I couldn't get warm.

When I went to sleep at night, I would think to myself, "If I only had a warmer coat and just kept it on all day, I could keep warm." It was crazy. Instead of dreaming of graduating and becoming Miss Washington, I was dreaming of coats and staying warm. I would also dream of peace.

The world was too loud, the days too long; there were too many voices, too many people, and too many places to be. Before, I could shut myself away with my books and the world would fade into the silence. I didn't have that luxury (or for me, the necessity) now. I needed quiet time or my brain started to overload. That's what was happening.

OVER THE EDGE

At the beginning of my senior year, I had to make the very agonizing decision to quit math. I say agonizing because I didn't want to quit, I felt I had to in order to keep my vow to never get a grade less than an A. I had made it through more years of math than I ever thought possible, and I was proud that I had conquered my worst subject. But by my senior year, I was slipping in all areas of my life and math slipped with me. I found myself totally unable to grasp the necessary elements of Calculus. By the end of the first quarter of the year, there was a good chance that I would probably get a D out of my math class.

I had come to believe that if I worked hard enough at school, I could do just about anything. I not only took mainstream courses, I got A's out of them. When help from my teacher and tutoring from my stepfather didn't help my math grade, I had to admit I was fallible. It was the first time in six years that I truly admitted to myself that there was something beyond my reach, that I was disabled.

To make up for what I felt was an inadequacy in math, the following trimester I signed up for a class which would prove to be my downfall. It was an optional class called College English. I didn't need to take any more English, I had fulfilled my requirements. But I felt I had to make up for my failure in math. I was going to take this College English class and show everyone that I could be as smart as they were.

English, although not quite as difficult for me as math, had its own complications. Spelling and sentence structure were two of my most dreaded tasks. I found it difficult to take essay tests or even to write an essay. If asked for an essay, I could recite it to you with no problem, but it was as though trying to write it during a test or in class made the information get stuck somewhere between my brain and my pen.

I couldn't type very well at the time and nearly every assignment and paper for this class needed to be typed. I had barely made it through typing class. The only reason I did get through it at all was due to the fact that I had a teacher who was more interested in my grasping the skill than in my taking timed tests. She made alternatives in the classroom available to me and I passed the class, but my skills were low.

I was unable to detect my own spelling errors, and I took forever just to write a one-page essay. It was obvious from about the fourth week on that I shouldn't have attempted to take this class. I had done fine in English before, but this was an honors class, and I was not in that league. I knew this, but I refused to quit the class. I had a good teacher and I thought I could get through.

By the second quarter of my senior year I was at the depth of my depression. My stamina for studying was down, and I was achy and tired in the mornings. When I went to the library at lunch time, the noise would distract me and depression seemed to loom over my head. The bell would ring and I would realize I had five books in front of me and very little work shown on my paper.

This was not good timing. I had achieved grades worthy of an A on the assignments in English up to this point. But now I was doing the final assignment, which was weighted heavier than all other assignments, and I couldn't pull myself together.

I kept trying to push myself but I was a broken person, there was nothing left to push. I barely eked out a report and hired a typist to type my report. I handed it in and waited for my grade. I handed in a report that was only the minimum amount of pages and I knew it wasn't very good. I needed help. Help in the class, help in my life.

I received a B on my report and a B in the class. I thought my other assignments would bring me up to an A minus, but I was under by just a few points. Before the class ended, I asked the teacher what my grade was. He said, "You have a B," and I broke down right in front of him. This was a class I didn't even need to take, a report I wouldn't have had to do. I asked him if there was a chance to bring up my grade. He said, "No," and I cried even more.

In my head I knew there probably wasn't anything he could do about my grade. I was crying not to gain sympathy but because I was out of control. Most people in my position would have been happy to get a B. My reaction shows how much importance good grades were in providing my sense of value. That B meant that I would not be second in my class. Once again, I had failed to meet my self-imposed standards, just a couple of months before graduation. I had promised myself that this wouldn't happen.

I was in such a panic when I left his room. I went to my social studies teacher and asked him what my grade was. He said, "Well, you have two A's and one B, but the B was the bigger test so you are close to getting a B." I started crying again. How could that be? I had done all the assignments, had done well on all the tests, and had been in class everyday. How could it be that with two A's and a B that I was getting a B?

I ended up with an A from his class, barely. But it became very clear to me just how far I was slipping, or had slipped, from the standards I had set. I was in a state of burnout. In the state that I was in, all I could focus on was the fact that not only did I fail myself in math and English, but now I was no longer second in my class. At some point, I knew I wouldn't be valedictorian, so being second highest had come to be my goal. Now, even that was impossible.

I look back on this incident and realize that I was over-reacting. I also realize that most people would find it difficult to sympathize with a person who has received only two B's. But getting A's had been the focal point of my life for years. Now they seemed to be slipping away from me. I can remember sitting across from my vice principal and asking him if there was anything I could do to retake my English class or redo the report. I knew there probably wasn't anything he could do. Maybe that isn't why I went to him. Maybe I just wanted someone to understand how desperately I had tried to make it, how long I had disguised my differences, and how hard I had to work to keep up. Maybe that's all I wanted, for someone to say, "It's okay, you have made it, we accept you."

But instead, everyone just asked, "What is it you want, Shari? Why is a B such a big deal, Shari? Do you want to be everything, Shari?" I can remember their faces. They looked at me with flat expressions and watched me fall apart.

No hand on my shoulder, nothing. All I really wanted, was for someone at my school to put a hand on my shoulder and tell me it would be all right. Is that so much to ask? Instead, I was just looked at as a girl who wanted and needed it all.

The last quarter of school I took only four classes instead of my usual six. I went to three classes in the morning and then came back for my leadership class and cheerleading in the afternoon. There was days I didn't even bother to return for my afternoon class.

With all the major sports completed for the year, the cheerleaders weren't making posters anymore and many of our duties were over. I had lost my drive in everything, including cheerleading, so unless we were doing something important, I didn't go. Everyone on the squad was wondering what was wrong with me. I couldn't admit to them that I felt like I was having a nervous breakdown.

In May of that year, shortly before graduation, a friend from the pageant set me up with a young man on a blind date. We got along well and began dating steadily. On one hand this was good, I wanted to have someone who liked me. The bad part was that I was extremely vulnerable. He was good looking and older; he took control and manipulated all situations. I wanted to be liked so much that I couldn't see how unhealthy this was. I was so weak from life that I couldn't get out of the relationship.

I think it suffices to say that I made mistakes in this relationship, my greatest one was sticking with it. I needed so much that I was willing to be controlled, and even used, just to get love. I was sacrificing my beliefs and my self-esteem to have someone like me.

I was voted "Most Likely To Succeed," and "Best Dressed" at our Senior Awards Breakfast, but I sat alone at the end of my table. I had been nominated for Homecoming Queen at the beginning of the year, but by the end of the year I wasn't even going to attend our senior ball or our graduation party. I was checking out early. I felt school had nothing left for me. I was bitter from the fight.

During our awards assembly, I came in late and sat by myself. The choir sang, but I was not with them; I wore a suit, my hair was done, and I looked much older than everyone else. Inside I felt like an old woman.

I did not stand when they called valedictorian and salutatorian; I stood when they called fourth in her class, Miss Shari Rusch. As I stood in front of my school, I looked at everyone and felt that I was separate from my classmates, that I didn't belong. It had always been that way; I was different. I was sad, but it was over now. I was ready to be done with all of it.

I stood to accept my Masonic Award Scholarship, and my Pageant Scholarship. But when the last scholarship award had been given I thought I had been called for the last time. Then I heard them announce, "The last and final award for today is the ASB Award, the award voted by the senior class for most outstanding student." I hadn't allowed such an honor to cross my mind. I knew I was up for it, my picture was in the annual with the other nominees, but other than that I tried not to think about it.

When they called my name, I was totally surprised. I walked up and accepted the award, but couldn't truly feel the honor that I was receiving. I was proud that my senior class thought so much of me that they would give me such an award, but at the same time I wondered why I never knew anybody liked me.

Graduation day came. It was the only day of my senior year I was looking forward to. Not because of the ceremony, but because graduation meant that my jail sentence (as I considered my school years) was over. I put on my gown and honor cords over a new blue dress that my mom had bought for me. It was a relief, and it was emotional for me and my family.

At the end of the ceremony, I gave my honor cords to a very special person, my resource room teacher from first grade. I felt is was important for Mrs. Schlosser to know she had made a difference in my life.

Rather than going to my graduation party, I went home. The next day I went to California with my mom and spent the next week sleeping. Most of the trip, we didn't even leave our room. I was that tired. My body had been tight and controlled, my mind like a robot for the last fifteen years. It was as if the springs of my body and mind had reached their stress points and were popping out in every direction.

My mom took me away for a week because I needed to have a little down time before I left for the Miss Washington pageant. I had less than seven days before I needed to leave. I needed more than seven days to put myself together, but that is all we had.

OVER MY FEET

I have always been an avid follower of ice skating. I sit on the edge of my seat through every move when watching competitions. At the 1988 Winter Olympics, Debbie Thomas had just completed the final competition against Katerina Witt. She had fallen and had several problems during the program as she tried to win the gold medal. When she stepped off the ice, the cameras and microphones were in her face immediately and they asked, "Debbie, what happened?"

She said, "Two things. First, I'm still alive and second, I just didn't feel over my feet tonight." She also commented that being the last performer made her nervous.

Her words described exactly how I felt when I was finished with the Miss Washington competition. Although the gravity of the situation was decidedly different, it was a competition all the same. I too was the last competitor to perform in each area of competition in the pageant.

I was one of 22 girls. Most of the other girls had been in pageants before so they knew the ropes. I, on the other hand, was a babe in the woods. I came in wide-eyed and watched as people laid out their territory.

For a person who required quiet to put her thoughts together I was in the wrong place. From the moment I arrived, it was non-stop, here, there, rehearsals all day long, and constant chaperones. I was nervous, scattered, and overwhelmed.

The only time I truly felt in balance and at ease with myself was when I sang. Otherwise, I asked myself, "Why am I doing this?"

I walked away from the pageant saying, "I am still alive." I had an interesting experience, scholarship money, and the non-finalist talent award. I knew then I would never run again.

I came home, unpacked, and started to cry. I cried for the next five months, maybe more. Sure, I was sad about the pageant, but it wasn't just that - it was everything. It was summer. There was no more noise, no place to go, nothing I had to do, no test to take. The hiding was over, high school was behind me. A major accomplishment had been achieved but there was no joy.

Every tear I hadn't cried over the last six years came out in a wave that wouldn't stop. I went to doctors to see if I was physically ill, but there was nothing physically wrong with me. This was a breakdown.

Before this, I could keep my emotions in check; not anymore. I cried in the shower and cried in the middle of my room.

While everyone else was looking forward to college and basking in the light of being a high school graduate, I spent most of that summer alone. College was the last thing I wanted to hear of or think about.

During my senior year I applied to only one college. I didn't rush to get applications, I didn't call colleges to find out their deadlines. While everyone else was rushing around, asking each other which college they were going to attend, I was listless. I had once dreamed of going to an Ivy League school, but I knew I couldn't leave home now. I was sick. Fortunately it all worked out, and I was accepted at the college of my choice.

I decided on the University of Washington because my sister was there and it was close to home. I decided to go through the sorority rush and pledge a sorority house, because it's what my sister had done. It didn't require thought - it was easy.

I should have been happy. After all, by finishing high school I had already accomplished more than had ever been expected of me. And here I was starting college. But each one of these major decisions that I muddled through reflected how tired and depressed I was. I couldn't think about the future, I could barely manage to get through each day. If I had thought about it at all I would have waited a year to go to college, and I would have gone to a smaller school, perhaps a community college, to avoid the large classes. But I couldn't think.

At the end of the summer, I went through rush and ultimately decided on joining the same sorority house that my sister had pledged. After I pledged, my life was like a whirlwind. I moved into the sorority house, which was my first time living away from home. It was very hard leaving with all my boxes. When I walked out the door of my mother's house, I felt more lost than ever.

I began to live a very different life. There were parties and activities all the time. I was living with close to a hundred girls and there was always something going on. I ate with these people, slept on a sleeping porch with three other people, and even studied with them. Literally, there was nowhere to go where there wasn't somebody. It was "community" everything.

I liked all the girls, but the constant noise and commotion wasn't good for me. I can't concentrate with other people in the room or stay up late and still do well in early morning classes. I knew my limits and found living in the sorority house to be very difficult.

I was fatigued and tired all the time. I was trying to adjust to college life, a sorority, and a school of approximately 36,000 people. It's no wonder I was tired; I could never let down my high level of concentration. I was always forced to tune out the noise of so many people.

I no longer had the luxury of coming home to a quiet empty house and cleaning to relieve my stress. The cleaning was done by hired help. I actually used to volunteer to do things in the kitchen because I needed my little patterns and rituals back again.

There was one place where I could find peace. I used to go down to the laundry room and shut myself in the closet. Yes, it is a little unusual but it was the quietest place in the house. I used to go down there every other day or so and work on a song or practice a speech. Believe me, everyone thought I was a little strange, but I had to do what worked for me; and if that meant standing in a laundry closet to collect my thoughts, I was going to do it.

One of the things that amazed me most about the sorority and college life was the lack of sleep that everyone seemed able to function on. I was a person who used to go to bed at 9:30 p.m. and get up at 4:00 a.m. to begin studying. Now everything was changed. I could go to bed at 9:30; but since 99 percent of the house didn't go to bed until midnight, the noise in the hall kept me up until at least midnight, too. I either had to stay up with everyone or try to sleep with noises all around me.

All of my patterns had changed. Everything was out of order: the time I slept, the time I ate, what I ate, the amount of noise and the activities that made up my life. I was not adjusting well.

I survived the sorority activities, but school was a whole different story.

I found myself sitting in classes with up to 850 people. I was just one of the masses. The professor looked like a little ant down on the floor, and his writing illuminated on the overhead projector was hard to read. More importantly, I found it hard to hear what he was saying and to concentrate on the information given in the lecture with that many people in the room.

I took only twelve credit hours that first quarter because I knew I would need more time to adjust and cope with the work load. My stepdad walked me through the registration phase, but my parents couldn't be with me every day as I faced the multitude of people, numbers, and buildings. Rod couldn't help me find my rooms, fill out forms, write my essays, or read the numerous books that I had to read. I was on my own.

I was taking introductory psychology, drama, and women's studies classes. Not a particularly heavy load, which was good for the state of mind I was in and the degree of learning problems I had, but still it was obvious from the beginning that the study skills I had in high school had to be intensified and refined. From the first day at college, I was working harder and longer hours, especially on reading. Even with all this I found it hard to keep up with my coursework.

I don't think the courses were too hard for me or that the work load was too heavy, it's just that everything in my life was different. I never had enough time to myself, I felt "spacey" and unsure of where I was most of the time. I got lost often, and I felt scattered and stressed when I finally made it to my classes. Often by the time I got to my classes, there wasn't a front row seat available, so I had to sit in the back and try to understand what was being said.

I wanted help but found that when I tried to go to the professors' offices, I would get lost. Then if and when I did get there, I felt pressured to hurry and get my questions over with because there were other people waiting behind me. I needed more instruction, more time to adjust, but there wasn't any.

My fragile mental state didn't help my ability to cope. I still found myself crying, depressed, and overly sensitive to small problems. Life itself felt incredibly heavy and frightening. I felt numb, unmotivated and in a mental anguish that I can't quite describe. I faked smiles, humor and laughs but all I really wanted to do was sleep.

My only relief was when I went home to my downstairs bedroom and stayed in my own bed. I often went home on the weekends. I missed many of the sorority activities that were arranged for the pledges to get to know each other. Without realizing it, I was isolating myself again. To me it was survival.

At some point, I had lost a lot of my motivation for school. I still worked as hard, but I just didn't go as far. Because of the size and noise of the school, I found that my learning problems were more pronounced than in high school. Had my mind, soul, and body been working together, I could have gone into college and done much better. In fact, in later classes when I was healing from my breakdown, I did much better. College wasn't impossible for me, it's just at that time I was too separated inside to feel the kind of single focused drive I needed to be successful at school.

ANSWERS

In the women's studies class, we covered women's issues of all types. So far, I have not had a class that made me think quite as hard about subjects that affect me and all other women on a day to day basis. The key word is "think." I didn't agree with everything they said. In fact, I disagreed at times, but being raised with divorce, in a single parent household, with a mom who worked full time and having watched my mom deal with men in business and personal circumstances, made me want to learn more about myself and the issues that affected me.

I was in a bad relationship at the time and was wondering why I allowed people to treat me as they did. When did that become okay? It wasn't okay for an employer to treat my mother badly, it wasn't okay for my mom's husband to treat her badly, so why had it become okay for me to be treated badly in relationships?

I took the class because my sister had recommended it. I walked out with a sense of self I didn't have before. I became a feminist in the sense that I wanted to live a different life from the one I had seen my mom live. I wanted better relationships than the one I was in. I no longer would be complacent and without respect for myself. Shortly after completing the course, I broke up with my boyfriend and vowed that I would no longer date people who wouldn't treat me with respect. I stuck to my word.

I loved this class. I participated in discussion groups with a passion. I read all the books that were required for the class several times.

I had an A in my quiz section (discussion group) because I would come to class totally prepared, ready to talk about what I had learned. To me, this was what college was all about. You don't take in the information and accept it, you think about it and form your own opinion. My other classes were dry by comparison.

The fact that I had an A in my discussion group and quiz section and that I read all the materials and turned in all my assignments made it even more shocking when I flunked the first test.

It was not because I hadn't studied the material. I was totally prepared. It's just that this was my first essay test in college. I had taken only a few essay exams in high school. It was also a timed test of fifty minutes. It would have never been enough time to untangle the tangles that formed in my brain when the teacher's aide said, "begin."

The way the room was built made each step, each dropped pencil, each whisper, echo. This was one of my smaller rooms, and yet the noise seemed deafening. Every ten to fifteen minutes the aide would go to the board and write down the amount of time that was left. Each time I looked up, I'd get distracted and become unable to concentrate. I had all the information and could express it verbally in class, but under pressure it felt like all the information was unreachable and unwriteable.

When my discussion group leader handed back the tests, she asked me to stay after class to receive my paper in private. I looked at my paper and saw the "F" on it. She thought there must have been some mistake, but there wasn't. I told her I had learning problems and that I choked on the test. She knew from discussion group that I had studied, so she referred me to one of the professors for help. I ended up passing the class and I got a tremendous amount of information from it, but I learned from that first test that I needed help. I could not conquer college on my own.

After that test, I began looking for help. Any kind of help from anybody. I thought surely in this school of 36,000 there must be help for someone like myself. There was no sign, no billboard, no card in the student union building, no information given at orientation. I called every number I could find. I even called the directory of the university, the information line, and asked for their help in finding this place that I knew had to exist. Each time I called, they said there was no such thing. Each number they did give me was incorrect.

On one occasion when I called the information line for help, I told them what I was looking for, explained my problem in full, and they came up with a number. I called the number and a woman answered. She said, "Yes, this is a disabled student service." I then described my problems with learning to her and asked her if I could get help. She asked, "How old are you?"

I answered, "Eighteen."

She said, "Well, we do take people up to the age of 19."

I thought that was odd considering that the average age of students in college is getting higher and higher. If it takes four years to complete school, and you start when you are 18, that would mean that you only get one year of help.

I asked, "What do people do to get help after they are 19?"

"We can refer you to the psychiatric department of the university at that point."

I sat in silence for a moment contemplating her words. I thought to myself, "You're right, after a year or more of trying to get help, I will need a psychiatrist's help." I determined that this was probably not the office I was looking for.

I continued my search during the next year and came up with nothing. By that summer, I was ready to drop out of school. I saw little hope of making the grades I expected from myself, and I knew I wouldn't be able to keep up for another three years without help.

What a change this was! I was actually asking for help openly, which I had seldom done before. I was willing to get help through an organization or even a resource room set up, if there was such a thing. Here was a person who dreaded the thought of separation and now I was actually asking for it. I was no longer concerned with looks. My burnout phase with school had brought me to the point where I couldn't worry about the trivial, it was my survival in school that was most important. And if that meant a resource room, I would have used it.

While looking for help with my learning problems, I continued making changes in my personal life. When I was in high school I had managed to make good decisions about alcohol despite what was often an intense need to fit in and be part of the party. I soon realized that as much as I wanted to fit in, as much as I wanted to have something remove any hurt that I had inside, alcohol didn't stop my pain, it just hid it for a while. In the bargain I lost control of myself and the situation around me. This is not how I wanted to live my life. By the time I reached college, alcohol was very accepted and accessible. I was overwhelmed and had a lot of personal issues that I was dealing with at the time. It seemed like a perfect solution. Take a drink and you will fit in. Despite it's acceptance, I didn't feel right about what I was doing. I knew in my heart that drinking or any other form of abuse was just a way to hide. It didn't solve the problems that I faced. It didn't take long for me to decide that I would never drink again. I started bringing soft drinks to parties and soon I just stopped going to them. It wasn't easy to buck the system. It wasn't easy to not be part of the crowd, but I looked at the people around me, the way that they acted under the influence and I knew that I didn't want to live my life like that.

In order not to eat, drink or sleep my pain away, I began to realize what I had always known deep inside. I needed to go for counseling. My mom urged me and urged me until finally I took the hardest steps of my life, into the office of a counselor. My mom wanted me well; I wanted to be well, I just didn't want to face all my pain. I didn't want to rehash the past.

My counselor was wonderful. I learned to talk to her about my dad, my stepsister, school, relationships and everything else. Things came out from every corner; emotions I had previously hidden came flowing out. When I came out of her office every week, I felt like a truck had run over me. I couldn't see that I was making progress at first. There was so much pain from all the years of hiding that I couldn't see beyond my emotions to the healing that would come.

But the healing did come. Getting it out was the hardest thing I ever did, but once it was out, the most amazing thing happened. I didn't have to run anymore. I started to feel freedom!

The first day that I entered counseling, I went in very composed. This wasn't going to shatter me, I wasn't going to lose control. I started to tell the counselor about my life. She listened intently as I described the horror of the suicide, the brokenness that I felt about my dad and the divorce. She said, "That's really awful, Shari, but the interesting thing is that you said it all with a smile on your face." She said, "You can cry here, Shari. You don't have to keep a stiff upper lip." I broke down right then and there and from that point on, I couldn't hold the tears back.

At the end of our first session, she handed me a weight. A huge piece of metal that was far too heavy for me to hold.

She said, "Shari, I want you to put that weight out in front of you and hold it with your arms extended." I thought, "This lady is crazy. I can't possibly hold this weight for more than a few seconds."

Once more, she told me to hold it out. I did, but I thought my arms would break. She started to talk as I held the weight. She said, "How does it feel to hold the weight?"

I said, "Awful; it hurts."

"How long can you hold it?"

"Not much longer." I then dropped it on the floor.

"Now what do you feel?" "Relief."

She said, "When you let go of the weight of the world, you will feel relief. When you stop taking responsibility for all that has gone wrong in your life and realize that your mom and dad and stepsister made decisions and that their decisions were not your fault, they just affected you, you will feel relief. Take the weight off your shoulders; it isn't your fault."

COMING BACK

After I started my counseling, several things happened. First of all, I started to come back to life again. From whatever depths I had slipped into, I was coming back. Second, I met a wonderful man, Dave. I had stopped dating for a while and was using the time to take care of myself. Maybe earlier I would have felt that I didn't deserve this person. Now I was ready to allow someone to care for me.

He came into a rehearsal for a show that I was in, and within a few weeks he sent me flowers. Two days after I received the flowers, we had our first date.

I had written a list of the things that I wanted a man to be many months before meeting him. As I think back on that long

269

list, I knew then that he had all of those traits. He was different from the other men I had dated. On our first date, I decided that I didn't want to hide anymore. Not in any way. On that lunch date, whether appropriate or not, I told him my whole life story from beginning to end. I was done before our entrees arrived. I thought it was better that he finds it all out now. If he can't take it, then I won't go out with him anymore.

Dave got an earful before the first course and I waited to see his reaction. Instead of asking what I had done to cause all of this or what was wrong with me that made me have such a difficult life, he said, "It is a shame that you had to go through that, it must have been very hard." He left it open so I could continue to talk, but that was all I needed to know.

Our first meeting was just the beginning. He saw me through counseling and recognized the need for it. He would even have gone with me if I wanted him to. He seemed to understand me so well and accepted me without reservation.

Dave had never suffered from learning problems. None of his family members had learning problems. So how was I to tell this new person in my life that I have learning disabilities, that I want to change the world by giving speeches on the subject, and at the same time get my college degree?

Dave may not have known much about learning problems or my dreams, but he listened and he learned. He was working as a sales representative by day and at night he was moonlighting as my "resource room teacher."

Not long after meeting him, I began taking a class about animal behavior. Towards the end of the course we had an assignment which involved figuring out which direction a bird would go if it were held in a cage with the light turned off for a certain length of time and then released to fly. The whole problem was rather complicated and I never fully understood which way that bird would fly. I remember Dave and I sitting together on my living room floor. He would explain the problem to me and I would just start to get it and then, boom! It was gone. I would have it one day but not the next. Dave stuck by me, trying to teach me. I never did get it. I'm lousy with directions anyway. If I were the bird (with my problems), I would have never left my cage.

I didn't get the problem right but Dave was helpful and understanding when it came to school. He did everything possible to encourage me.

More than that, he helped me with life. I was a very fragile person when I met him. I was not completely stable, but working on it. The world seemed big and overwhelming. Dave helped to break it down for me. Just as Rod helped my mom with filling out forms and adding figures on a ledger, Dave encouraged me to get credit cards, a checking account and to use a bank machine. These were things I swore I never would do. Life was already so complicated.

I was crippled by simple necessities of life. Book learning was all I had been able to cope with up to this point, but Dave knew that there were life skills that I would need to have to be able to survive in the world. These simple life skills were just the beginning. If I didn't understand something, he taught me how it worked. This new knowledge of the world was frightening, but it made me feel stronger and more capable.

When I went through depressions, he was with me. When I had nightmares, he would listen when I talked about them. And when I was afraid, he would console me and encourage me to keep going.

He is a very strong Christian, and he introduced me to a whole new world of prayer and Christian music. Music could always reach me in a place that words couldn't. It was this new kind of music that smoothed out my rough edges. It gave me something to hang on to. He encouraged me to pray out loud, to pray with him and to trust in God in a way that I hadn't ever done before. Although it was a gradual process, I soon learned to rely on my faith as a way to recover from some of my depression and worry. Each part was a step to my becoming whole again.

Previously, people had tried to keep me down in relationships or control me and keep me from reaching my potential. Dave was showing me how to depend on myself to get through the day. He encouraged me to be the best that I could be and to move forward with my dreams and goals in all areas of my life.

A few months after I met Dave, I was to give up my crown and pass it on to another young woman at the yearly pageant. For me, this was going to be a very important night. I had prepared a slide show showing what I had done on behalf of learning disabled and physically disabled people that year. I wanted my Dad to be there and I asked him to come. He said he would try, but when the night came, he never showed up.

I was his daughter. I wanted to make him proud; that is what I always wanted. When I stood out on the stage and thanked everyone for being a part of my life and for their support, knowing he wasn't there made me feel like a lost little child again. This was only one of the many instances when I said to myself, "If he loved me, he would have come."

I decided that night at the pageant that I wasn't going to call him, I wasn't going to beg, I wasn't going to be the lost child anymore. When I made that decision, there were no limits. I didn't say I would not see him again for a certain amount of time. I just said to myself, "You aren't going to call him anymore. Let him call you and then see where you can go from there. Let him take the initiative this time." For a long time I expected a call, for a long time I waited.

The call never came.

The only information that I received about him was from my sister. She would visit with him and then come back and tell me how much he missed me. I thought if he missed me so much, he would pick up the phone and call me. She never had an answer for that. When she did answer me it was with, "That's just the way Dad is."

As time went on, she would ask me to go with her to meet with my father. I always said, "No." I felt sure that if he truly wanted me there he would call and ask me to come. Once again, he never called.

I did not see my father for a year and a half. I did not sit and lament the loss. I soon learned not to wait for the phone to ring. I did not do it to punish him. I did it because I was a grown woman still wishing for her daddy. I knew I would ruin relationships and ruin myself if I didn't get over it and figure out how to deal with the father that I had, not the father that I longed for.

I grew up in that year and a half. Counseling was a roller coaster. I had it out with all my demons in those sessions. Even though it was only my counselor and I in the room, I talked to my father, cried for my stepsister, and cried for the loss of childhood I had experienced at the hands of life.

If I hadn't ever said it before, I was saying it every time I went to counseling, every time I went to school in the morning with depression looming over my head, I was saying that I wanted to live, I wanted to be happy, and I wanted to laugh again. Something was happening inside of me. It was no longer the good grades that were important, it was no longer the cheer sweater or the awards, it was no longer the plaques or crowns or people who liked me. It was life that I wanted now.

Before I had just gotten by, now I wanted to live life the way I thought it could be lived. Not a utopia, I knew that was not realistic, but a life that was more up than it was down, and a life where even the downs are not so bad because you know you won't be there forever.

I wanted to have it all happen at once. I wanted to live a new life right away, but the climb out of my bottomless pit was slow. Yet, with each step, I found a new answer.

CHAPTER
17

After the second quarter of my freshman year, I moved out of the sorority house and became a "Townie." I still participated in sorority activities, but I lived at home. I moved out because I could no longer cope with the noise or the late nights. For me to function in school, I had to have a quiet place to study and a place to sleep where I could go to bed early. Moving was just one of the positive steps I was taking to put myself back together. I had the support of my family, and peace.

That summer I continued my quest to find some help at the University of Washington. I was getting desperate. The new school year was coming and I was wondering how much longer I could continue without help. After making a few more phone calls with little progress, I turned to my Mom and Rod and said, "I can't be the only one searching for help. I can't be the only one who is ready to drop out because she can't find the services she needs!"

I became frustrated and angry. Why should a college education be out of my reach? Why should other people be able to have this, but not me? If I'm willing to do everything to help myself, then why can't I get some assistance? I wondered if they didn't make the information about services available because they didn't want disabled students to attend the university. If they don't make it available, many people would think it's not possible for them to go to a university, so they won't even apply. Was it survival of the fittest?

One phone call later, the University of Washington information operator finally gave me the correct number. Within a week, I was sitting in the office of the Director of Disabled Student Services.

On the way down to her office I turned to my mom and said, "Maybe I should not have dressed up, maybe I should have worn my glasses." I had worked so hard at not looking disabled, or thinking disabled, that I thought maybe they will look at me and say, "Sorry, you have to look and act a certain way before we will help you." However, the director looked beyond my outward appearance. She knew that you could not recognize a person with learning disabilities just by looking at them. She was a warm, kind person and I knew immediately that she was there to help me make it through school.

I had tried not to look the part of a learning disabled person and had been able to outsmart the public school system for so long, I began to worry that maybe if I was tested again, they wouldn't be able to tell what was wrong with me.

I soon found out that no clever tactics on my part could hide my disabilities from a test designed to find a learning disability if it existed. I soon had a fifteen page report from the Washington Association of Children With Learning Disabilities to prove that.

The test results made me eligible for the program and the services

275

that were available to me through the university. These services included a list of students and their major or expertise. I could call these people at any time to obtain help in a certain subject. I would have longer testing times. I could put my answers directly on the test rather than filling out a computerized answer sheet, which in my experience resulted in my answers being put in the wrong column. I would be able to take my test in a room either by myself or with a proctor. The room would be silent and I would be able to concentrate. I would receive free lecture notes and a student in each of my classes would be assigned to help me by going over my notes with me or by giving me a copy of her notes to supplement what I could do on my own. I could get a front row seat reserved in my classes if that was necessary for me to be able to see the overhead, hear, and get a good tape recording of the class.

The disabled student service would have people tape my text books for me; but more than that, the director described a program I had never heard of before. She told me that once I was tested and eligible for the Disabled Student Service, I could apply for books on tape from the national and state Libraries for the Blind and Physically Handicapped. She said, "At least through their program, learning disabled college students with documentable learning problems can get books on tape simply by applying for them." It was the best thing that ever happened to me.

Through the Libraries for the Blind, I was able to get books of every description on tape. Not just text books, but leisure reading books and magazines if I wanted them. Each month or so, I would receive new catalogs of titles and all I had to do was use the borrower numbers that were assigned to me for each library. I would call and leave my title requests on a tape recorder. In a week or so, I would receive the books. There was no charge for this or any other service. All I had to do to return the books was to turn the label on the front of the tape carton over and put them in my mail box.

My mom and I couldn't believe it! Here was this wonderful service and we didn't even know it. I kept thinking what a shame it was that students who really wanted an education might think they couldn't have it. Here were the tools that would give them an equal opportunity.

From that time forward, I made a point of talking about the services I received at the college level and telling my audience that, by law, all schools are to have services like these available to students. It is imperative that kids know what is available to them and that services such as the ones that I receive are properly funded and supported. I want students, parents and teachers to know that people with learning disabilities can continue to achieve beyond high school. They can go to college if that is their choice. We should encourage students with all ranges of disabilities to seek higher education.

As I look back on the time that it took to find the services that I needed and the tremendous effect that they had for the good once I found them, it saddens me that the services available to me in college were not in the public secondary schools nor are they available in most of the schools that I visit from day to day. Students who can't get through high school are not going to make it to college. But with the proper tools and skills, they could make it. Books on tape, longer testing times to correct spelling and answers, oral tests, are just some of the things that we could do early on in our children's schooling to keep the learning disabled students from dropping out and get them on to college and a successful life.

By the end of the session, my mom and I were crying with gratitude. We were so happy to have found an answer; I am continually grateful for the workers at the disabled student service and those people around the nation who work at the Libraries for the Blind and other services for people with disabilities of all kinds.

With the service's help I was able to raise my grade point from a 3.2 to a 3.35 in a year and half. It doesn't sound like very much, but anybody familiar with grade points knows that going up is much harder than coming down. According to the tests that were done to determine my eligibility for the Disabled Student Service, with my disabilities I should only be able to achieve between a 1.5 and 2.0 Grade Point Average. Another assessment proven wrong.

In time, I found that there were many options for furthering my education if I just kept my eyes open. One of these options was finding that I could take a quarter off from the university and take classes at a community college where the class size would be smaller. And my credits would transfer! I found that the smaller classes were much better for me. The amount of noise and distraction was less, I could hear and see better, and consequently, I learned more and received better grades while still maintaining my status at the university.

When my mom and I left the disabled student service we had to walk over a bridge that led to the parking garage. As we walked, my mom looked ahead where you could see just a glimpse of the huge buildings and vast size of the campus. She looked at me and said, "Now I see why going here is so frightening to you. It is so big. You're doing what I was too afraid to do."

That same month, during the summer before my sophomore year, I sat down at the typewriter and didn't get up for a very long time. It was then that I wrote the first edition of this book.

After numerous speaking engagements for schools and service groups, I had been showered with requests for my story in written form. With a year and a half of speaking behind me and a little time off before school started again, I began writing my story.

Writing the first edition of my story answered some questions for me, this second edition has answered even more. Writing my story is like riding a roller coaster. I am tired and fatigued as I write because I hit the keys backwards, the screen blurs and the words don't come easily.

There were many days when I wanted to throw in the towel. There were nights when I have bundled up my manuscript in a folder convinced that I needed to get a professional writer to ghost write the story for me. "I'll say it, they'll write it." But the next day, I always decided to unbundle it and start again.

GETTING THE MESSAGE HEARD

When my first book was published and people began buying it, my public speaking career also took off. I went from place to place sharing my story locally on a volunteer basis.

These first two years of public speaking were my education, and what an education it was! When I first started speaking, I shook with fear behind the podium. The podium became my protection and I used it as such. Just in case the audience rioted, I was prepared. That is how little confidence I had in myself.

As did all the speakers I had seen, I wrote out my speech on note cards, but the writing was too small. Then I tried to memorize it word for word, but I tended to forget my speech under pressure. I also found that one small movement in the audience could disrupt my thought pattern to the point where I would lose my place in my memorized speech. I tried large outlines, written out and highlighted, and still I couldn't read it under pressure. I realized early on that notes were useless to me. I had to prepare my speech in advance and hope to God that nobody dropped something and distracted me.

In time, I learned that just as I had developed a high level of concentration at home with my books, or in class with commotion all around me, I did the same thing with speaking. Now I can stand in front of any audience and not see the distractions that at one time would have put my mind into a tailspin.

Once I had the concentration, I needed to work on retention of my material. I found that writing certain points, thoughts, or even the whole speech was helpful. Then to lock the information in, I would say it out loud in my hotel room or at home. Saying the words out loud was like reading a book out loud to myself. It would reinforce the information that was stored on the page or in my brain because I could hear it. To write it and read it was fine, but to say it meant the information was locked in.

I must emphasize the word repetition. Without it, even the most common point that I had made many times would not come out properly. I had to keep in constant contact with the information I was speaking on or the information got lost in my head.

Because I spoke without notes, I had nothing to fall back on. Because I couldn't memorize my speech, it meant that once I got up to the podium, I had to be spontaneous. Sometimes a story would be changed around, sometimes a story would be left out. Sometimes new material I wanted to add would show up, but I would say it somewhat differently than planned. Some days were easier than others.

With each speech, I gained experience and with that experience came an amazing change. When I started to trust my brain and myself a little more, when I gained a little confidence, I found that my brain put the points in order just as I had practiced. If I didn't panic, the stories came out in order and, in general, I looked like I was in complete control.

Yes, I eventually learned not to panic, but in the beginning stages of speaking I was a bundle of nerves. I put myself through turmoil before a speech, worrying and fretting about what to say and how to say it. If I had a speech on Friday, I began worrying and losing sleep the previous Sunday. By the time one speech was over, I started worrying about my next one.

Often, when a speech was over, I was so relieved, I didn't hear the applause. I was so self-critical, I would chastise myself for every little mistake. There were times when I would feel totally empty after a speech because I never allowed myself to fill up with anything. No applause or nice words could get through my barrier of self-doubt and worry.

One of my greatest fears from the very beginning was that I wouldn't be enough. It only took a few speeches to realize the amount of needs that existed in each audience that I spoke to. My old perfectionist attitude kept telling me that I should be able to save them all and have all the answers. The students, their parents, and the educators that I came into contact with were so hungry for answers, and I felt so inadequate to meet their needs, that it was just another reason to quit.

Well, I didn't quit. I just learned that I might not have all the answers and that was okay!

Besides the needs of my audiences, there was something else that I battled with. I used to be able to give my speech in twenty minutes because I would gloss over the toughest parts of my life. I had lived out my pain in counseling and with my family, and talking about it in front of strangers was not my idea of a fun

279

afternoon.

Talking openly about difficult, but relevant, parts of my story was a gradual process. Slowly but surely I allowed myself the time to bring out little bits and pieces as I was comfortable to do so. It was hard, but I knew that I had to be open and honest so that people could see the transition that took me from where I used to be to the present.

I asked myself many times, "Will I hurt someone if I say this?" "Will my message make people uncomfortable?" Maybe it would. But what if it will help someone understand how I got through it all? Then it is relevant and important for me to say. Now I can share without reservation whatever I need to. I can touch more people by being honest. Now I am real. Now the links to my story are all in place.

I might have thought that I was opening up to benefit other people, but speaking even about the difficult parts of my life helped me to heal, too.

Six years of speaking are now on my resume and I know in my heart that it has been the hardest and the most rewarding path that I could ever have chosen. I now travel extensively throughout the United States speaking at schools and at state, national and international conferences for students, educators and business people. It is my full-time career and I love it.

When I started public speaking at age eighteen, I was the same age as the kids and could be the daughter of most of the adults who sat in my audiences. When they heard my age, some would look at me, doubting my wisdom because of my youth. It took me a little while to realize that when I was standing up on that stage I had to forget my age and hope they would too. I needed to keep in check the emotion that goes hand in hand with my story. I needed to approach my story and my audience, no matter who they were, as an adult, and at the same time have the conviction and emotion in my speech that would move people to change. It was a hard balance to create at first, but it eventually became easier and easier.

I went into public speaking thinking that I could save the world. A few crossed arms later I realized that maybe I couldn't change everyone and everything. When I talk to administrators and teachers, some will embrace what I have to say and give their students hope for their futures. Others will want to legitimize the current treatment of their students by saying that I am one-in-a-million and that their students couldn't possibly achieve what I have.

At school assemblies, there are students who hug me, run to talk to me after the assemblies, and write me letters. But there are always those few who sit up at the top of the auditorium seats.

I notice them because they sit with their heads hung or hide behind a paper or a book. I used to be so discouraged by those I thought I wasn't reaching; then I would receive a letter from that girl or boy whom I thought wasn't listening, or the teacher whom I thought was hardened after so many years of struggling on behalf of kids, to say that I had touched them.

Sharing my story has changed me in so many ways - it has made me stronger. I used to think that when I stood stiff as a board and told my story without flinching or crying that I was strong. I used to think that if I could walk out of a school without being touched emotionally, that I was strong. But I know now that I am strong because I am touched by my audience. I do feel their joys and sorrows. I am just better at handling that load. I guess the bottom line is, I no longer carry the load alone. My faith in God has helped me to give some of the burden away.

I am not only touched by my audience and feel what they are going through, but I am much more in touch with what I feel. I have gone through periods of time in my speaking career, particularly in the beginning, where things got very serious. I thought I had to be serious to be taken seriously. I was afraid to let my sense of humor out for fear that people would not hear the urgency in my voice; that they wouldn't feel my commitment for making change. Instead I found just the opposite. As I slowly let my natural self come out and my sense of humor took over the content of my message, I realized that my story was easier for people to handle. They could take the lows as long as they were coupled with some laughter. I guess that is really what life is all about. Learning to laugh about the past makes the present a lot easier to deal with.

The real reward from speaking is the caring administrator, the effective teacher, the loving parent, and the smile from the kid in the front row. It's the letter from the boy who tried to commit suicide several times but is now turning his life around, the meeting with the anorexic young girl who is trying to learn how to heal, and the tough kid that you thought you didn't reach but comes up to ask you to sing in his rock band that weekend.

There are many rewards, but most importantly, there is the affirmation that my message is being heard and understood. The hugs from the elementary school children. The scrawled handwriting from a learning disabled child who had the courage to write despite her problems. The seven-page letter from a girl who suffers from agoraphobia, a disorder which makes her fear leaving her house, but who is now going to school two times a week. These things are my affirmations and my hope.

The pictures and the thank-you notes. The t-shirt that is presented by the school when my speech is over and the cheers that come when I put it on. The poem from a loving principal who heard my story. The resource room teacher who now believes her kids are going to make it. I take every one of them with me and keep them in my prayers.

My message has spanned beyond the resource room. The lessons I have learned and the friendships I have made have been with people who face all different kinds of challenges, not just learning disabilities.

From place to place on my travels I have seen the courage that it takes for developmentally or physically disabled persons to go to school every day when those around them, the "normal kids," seem to walk through life with ease and have little understanding of what life is like for others. I have heard their hopes and dreams for the future and I have also heard some say that they are afraid that they won't get there because, after all, they are disabled.

Maybe I too would have wondered just how far people could go if I hadn't lived it. I no longer wonder. I know that with love and support, with alternatives provided, with schools and systems of society that allow for differences among people that all of the kids that I meet can achieve their goals. I read slowly, others walk or move slowly, some even speak slowly but their value is no less. We all want jobs, we all want to achieve our goals and our dreams. We all want to be productive. With proper help, we can be.

The kids that I have met, their parents and their teachers want people to ask questions rather than stare, to provide opportunities rather than closed doors and to look upon those with challenges, whether hidden or not, as productive people with as much to offer the world as any other citizen.

I have been taught these valuable lessons from the children, young adults, parents and teachers that I have met on my travels. Thanks to Bart, Scott, Vangie, Holly, Adam, Tim, Angie, Jaime, Diane, Elizabeth, Jeff, Scott, and all of my other friends out there. You have kept me going. Your success and letters have fueled me to keep going as a speaker, writer, and person.

It is said that children are the future. Judging from the kids that I have met, the tough and the fragile, the bright and the different, I think that with a little love, we will be led by a wonderful new generation.

ADAM

Adam wrote me a letter the other day. He is now graduated from high school and has a steady job. More importantly to both of us was that with the money he makes from his job, he is paying for classes that will enhance his reading and speaking abilities. These were skills that he should have learned in high school; but he is not bitter. He is as sweet as ever. I know he is going to make it.

I recently asked Adam, "If you had the chance to tell the world something, what would it be?" Although he wrote me a three-page letter in response, I will paraphrase what he said with this one sentence: Prejudice of any kind, whether against race, color, or difference is painful and unfair and should never exist. I couldn't agree more.

ONLY THE BEGINNING

Four years ago on Father's Day, I began seeing my father again. One day I woke up and it was over. I was an adult. I was not the crying, needy child that I used to be. My pain had been healed with counseling, a wonderful man was in my life and I had a stepfather who I had come to trust and love. I no longer had to have my father's approval, I no longer was begging. I was now whole.

Without telling my father, I showed up at his Father's Day dinner with my sister. It was so uncomfortable that I was glad when the dinner came to an end. I was not uncomfortable because I hadn't seen him, I was uncomfortable because I realized that I had grown up. I was a different person now.

After that, we began meeting. Our first meetings were only with my sister. He would make arrangements with her and we would all meet together. At these meetings, my sister was highly uncomfortable and tried to keep the conversation going. My dad made an effort, it seemed, to initiate conversation. I tried to act involved but I couldn't help being distant. I had to find a new place for myself now. If I wasn't the little girl, who was I? One year passed and we began meeting without Shawn. It was around that same time that I received one of the first phone calls he had made to me in several years. I was sick and he called to see how I was doing. It meant the world to me.

I love him very much. He is my father. I came back to him because I wanted to try to know him and for him to know me. I wanted to have a relationship with him. The difference was that I came back into the relationship with no expectations. I no longer needed a daddy. I had found the missing love that I needed in Dave and Rod. I was no longer searching frantically to fill up the void. Without that pressure, I could start fresh with my father.

Since I began seeing my father again, we have never discussed our time apart, our differences or the past. We still have a way to go but we are able to speak better to each other with each passing meeting.

When David and I decided to get married, I asked my father to give me away. He walked me down the isle, the most healing steps we have taken in our whole lives.

I now talk to my dad once a week or every other week. The calls are not strained anymore and we say "I love you" at the end of the phone call. I don't know how it happened. One day it just came out. Now it sounds natural. I am proud of the growing relationship that I have with him.

Recently, my father came to see me speak for the first time since I began my career. After my speech, I sat down next to him and he put his hands on my back. I looked at him and he had tears in his eyes. I told my story to a crowd of strangers that night, but it was as if the only person I was speaking to was my father. I tried to explain all the years and all my differences in that one hour. I hadn't looked at my father during the entire speech for fear I would cry. I found my father that night and my father found me. He told me he was proud of me. I loved hearing those words.

My mom has now been happily married for ten years. Her company has grown from doing small mall productions to large statewide events and productions. Rod, my stepfather, recently retired from 30 years in education and is co-owner of their company.

When I was growing up, my mom would have liked to fix all my problems; sometimes she couldn't. It was during those times that she looked for an alternative. When she could fight off the bad guys, she did. And when she couldn't chase them away, she would hold me in her arms and say, "I love you Shari, it will be all right."

She has chased her demons as I have chased mine. She is no longer running scared. How did she get through all those years so successfully while in so much pain, always there for others but seldom for herself? I am extremely proud of her and would fight tigers to protect her. She would do the same for me.

Together, we found our way.

Then came Rod. He loved my sister, Mom and me without conditions. He came into our lives and brought a calming force and strength that made our lives settled.

He is a patient and kind man. He is as organized as my mom is creative. He does the books - she has the ideas. When we came into his life we were all a bit scattered. All frightened.

Especially me. He came into my life at the beginning of the break and saw me through to the healing.

He tutored me through school, he gave me encouraging words about school and about life, he was the calm voice that said it will be okay. He would always be there on important occasions. He would drop what he was doing in a flash if I needed a ride to school. He has driven hundreds of miles to get me to speaking engagements when I was afraid I would get lost. He has been the consistency, the fatherly love, the stabilizer of the last ten years.

Dave and I were married on June 18, 1988. We bought a house, adopted a kitten, and are living the life I always wanted to lead. He loves me and I love him in a way that I never believed was possible. He listens to me, respects me, encourages me and is the voice of comfort and reason when the world seems mixed up.

Some people say that marriage is hard, that in this day and age it is hard to keep it together. I don't think it will be for us. We waited over three years before we got married. I needed time to sort things out; he gave me that time. I learned to trust again, to believe that not all men would leave me; and I learned that marriages can last if both people try.

As a kid of divorce, I needed to heal. I did. Now there is no doubt in my mind that our marriage will last. Our priorities are God, family and our work, in that order.

A great deal of thanks goes to my family. All of them: Rod, my mom, Shawn, Dave, and my grandparents, Marguerite and Oscar Eyrikson. They have loved me through this whole process.

I am now a graduate of the University of Washington with a Bachelors of Arts degree in Psychology. My family knew which graduate I was at the ceremonies because I was doing hand springs down the aisle. Just kidding! You heard my gymnastics story didn't you? The truth is, I wanted to do hand springs down the aisle but knowing that I might hurt myself, I opted for a simple pomp and circumstance walk.

I am obtaining my teaching certification, and someday I will also get my masters in education. Maybe I will open a school someday where all students are shown alternative forms of learning and all are accepted.

No matter what, I will continue to speak, write and sing. I will continue to tell my story in the hope that other people will not only listen, but understand and make the changes happen. Everyone has the right to succeed, and it is our challenge to help each other, no matter how narrow the path or how long the road, or how bad the eyesight or hearing, how large the brace or wheelchair. No matter what the learning problem or obstacle a person may have to live with, we are all equal and deserve the chance to show the world that we can achieve.

□

Isn't it strange that captains and kings and clowns that caper in sawdust rings, and just plain folks like you and me and builders of our destiny, have each been given a bag of tools, a shapeless mass and a book of rules, and each must fashion ere time has flown, a stumbling block or a stepping stone.

R.L. Sharp

If you would like to write to Shari Rusch please send letters to:

Shari Rusch c/o Arc Press
P.O. Box 82627, Kenmore, WA 98028

ORDER FORM

	Price	Postage x Quantity	Quantity	Sub-Total
Stumbling Blocks to Stepping Stones (Book Only).............	12.00	2.00		
Stumbling Blocks to Stepping Stones "Book On Tape" (4 Audio Cassettes) ...	15.00	2.00		
Cassette Single including: **I Won't Cry Anymore & One Single Voice**	3.50	.50		
(written and performed by Shari Rusch)				
Package #1 including Book & Cassette Single	14.50	2.00		
Package #2 including "Book On Tape" & Cassette Single	17.50	2.00		
Package #3 including Book, "Book On Tape" & Cassette Single.............	27.00	3.00		

* Washington State residents must add a 6.5% sales tax to the Total Sales (do not include postage and handling when determining this tax).

Sub-Total: _____

State Tax (if applicable*): _____

GRAND TOTAL: _____

Make checks and money orders payable to Arc Press. No cash please. Make sure you have applied postage to each item you have ordered.

Shari Rusch c/o Arc Press
P.O. Box 82627
Kenmore, WA 98028

*** Make sure you have enclosed the correct address, order form and your check or money order. Mail to:

Please print clearly the name and address of the recipient.

NAME _____

ADDRESS _____

CITY _____

STATE _____ ZIP _____

CUT ALONG THIS LINE.

RECOMMENDED BOOKS

Anderson, Louie. *Dear Dad, Letters From an Adult Child.*
Markam, Ontario: Penguin Books, 1989.
A very personal look at what it is like to be the child of an alcoholic. Filled with humor, warmth and resolve to repair a broken parent/child relationship.

Buscalia, Leo. *The Fall of Freddie the Leaf.*
Henry Holt and Company, 1982.
This book is one of the most refreshing, insightful and yet simple views of the overwhelming issues associated with death. It is a perfect way to introduce the subject to children and will offer a new perspective to adults.

Haden, Torey L. *One Child.*
New York, New York: Avon Publishers, 1981.
I recommend all books by Ms. Haden. She is a phenomenal teacher who manages to reach the seemingly unreachable children and tells their stories with such understanding. Her stories are remarkable.

Morris, Harold. *Twice Pardoned.*
Pamona, California: Focus on the Family Publishing, 1986.
An ex-convict talks about life, mistakes and how he went from nothing to everything and is now changing the world for the better.

Peal, Norman Vincent. *The Power of Positive Thinking.*
New York, New York: Fawcett Crest, 1963.
I recommend all books by Dr. Peale. They are life changing books with a universal message that can be applied to any and all areas of life.

Peretti, Frank. *This Present Darkness.*
This book is a strong testimony to the power of prayer. His follow-up book, *Piercing The Darkness,* is equally inspiring.

Schlafly, Phyllis. *Child Abuse in the Classroom.*
Westchester, Illinois: Crossway Books, 1985.

Excerpts from official transcripts of proceedings before the U.S. Department of Education regarding the curriculum in our public schools.

Smith, Sally L. *No Easy Answers: The Learning Disabled Child at Home and at School.*
New York, New York: Bantam Books, 1979.

An excellent look at all aspects of learning disabilities through the eyes of the author who is a teacher, an administrator and a parent.

Somers, Suzanne. *Keeping Secrets.*
New York, New York: Warner Books, 1988.

An insightful look at the life threatening problems that are associated with being the child of an alcoholic.